J. Treib (Ed.)

Volume Therapy

Springer

Berlin
Heidelberg
New York
Barcelona
Hong Kong
London
Milan
Paris
Singapore
Tokyo

J. Treib (Ed.)

Volume Therapy

With 50 Figures and 26 Tables

With Contributions by

J.Boldt, D. J. Cole, F. Cortbus, M T. Grauer, A. Haass, H. Iro
E. T. Riley, K. W. Ruprecht, R. Schell, V. Scherer, W. I. Steudel
G. Stier, F. Waldfahrer

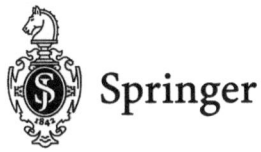 Springer

Johannes Treib, Priv.-Doz. Dr. med.
Universitätskliniken des Saarlandes
Neurologische Klinik
Kirrbergerstraße
D-66421 Homburg/Saar

ISBN-13: 978-3-642-64054-4   e-ISBN-13: 978-3-642-59621-6
DOI: 10.1007/ 978-3-642-59621-6

Springer-Verlag Berlin Heidelberg New York

Library of Congress Cataloging-in-Publication Data
Volume Therapy/Johannes Treib, editor. p. cm.
Includes bibliographical references and index.
ISBN 978-3-642-64054-4
1. Infusion therapy. 2. Blood plasma substitutes. I. Treib, J. (Johannes), 1965-.
RM170. V65 1999   615'. 39--dc21   99-42741

© Springer-Verlag Berlin Heidelberg 2000
Softcover reprint of the hardcover 1st edition 2000

Cover design: design & production, Heidelberg
Typesetting: Goldener Schnitt, Sinzheim
SPIN: 10702696   18/3134   5 4 3 2 1 0 – Printed on acid-free paper

Preface

Volume therapy or infusion therapy is used worldwide for the treatment of hypovolemia caused by surgical blood and plasma losses, trauma, burns, or infections. Interestingly, significant differences exist between countries regarding the use of plasma substitutes. In the United States, crystalloids and albumin are more popular, whereas in Europe artificial colloids such as hydroxyethyl starch are preferred. From an international perspective, it is notable that volume therapy using hydroxyethyl starch is an established therapy for the treatment of cerebral, retinal, otogenic, and peripheral circulation disorders in Germany. In other countries, crystalloids are mostly used to treat dehydration or hypovolemia, for example in brain stroke. In recent years, new data made it possible to overcome national differences and agree on an evidence-based, international consensus.

The efficacy of different plasma substitutes for a volume therapy lasting several days has not been sufficiently studied in the past. Long-term volume therapy of patients with cerebral perfusion disorders is an excellent model for studying the effects of artificial colloids in detail, because of the high doses of colloids that are administered. Through a comparison of commonly used plasma substitutes, we were able to show that significant differences exist between different colloids, for example in their effect on coagulation. After repeated infusion, hydroxyethyl starches that are difficult to degrade lead to an accumulation of large molecules that are difficult to eliminate. These large molecules impair factor VIII/von Willebrand factor. Easily degradable, medium, or low molecular weight hydroxyethyl starches, on the other hand, result in no clinically relevant changes in the coagulation system.

The adequate choice of plasma substitutes made it possible to extend the use of artificial colloids, for example in high-dose, hemodynamic volume therapy for the treatment of cerebral perfusion disorders. In the past, studies of hemodynamics in patients with acute stroke were limited to blood pressure, because measuring cardiac output was invasive and time-consuming. The thoracic bioimpedance method now allows for noninvasive, continuous measurement of cardiac output. Using this method, we studied the significance of hemodynamics for volume therapy by measuring the hemodynamic baseline of patients with acute stroke and compared these values with a control group matched for age and gender.

The improvement of hemodynamics and rheological parameters is a promising therapy approach for ischemic stroke because, due to the impaired autoregulation, the perfusion of the ischemic brain region depends on blood pressure, cardiac output, and rheological properties. Volume therapy attempts to increase cardiac output and blood pressure through an increase in cardiac preload and to improve rheological properties of the blood by decreasing plasma viscosity and erythrocyte aggregation. According to recent studies, hemodynamics is of decisive importance for volume therapy. The results of clinical hemodilution studies carried out so far suggest that a decrease in hematocrit during acute stroke will only result in clinical benefits, if hemodynamics is improved at the same time. The concept of isovolemic hemodilution, with the goal of improving microcirculation based on the decrease of blood viscosity alone, has not been shown to be effective in acute stroke. Our hemodynamic measurements showed that isovolemic hemodilution, contrary to hypervolemic hemodilution, does not result in an improvement of hemodynamics. In addition, bloodletting that was carried out too fast led to a brief worsening of hemodynamic parameters. Hypervolemic hemodilution therapy attempts to optimize hematocrit and stabilize cerebral perfusion through an increase in cardiac output and blood pressure. The administration of volume improves ventricular filling through the Frank-Starling effect and increases cardiac output through the increase in stroke volume without increasing heart frequency. The results of several multicenter studies confirm (within limits) the clinical effectiveness of this concept.

In addition, volume therapy is used to treat perfusion disorders in the fields of anaesthesiology, opthalmology, otorhinolaryngology and neurosurgery. Current review articles continued in this book give the reader an overview how volume therapy is applied in these specialties.

The limitation of reperfusion damage through a „plugging" of the capillary leak is another current therapeutic concept in volume therapy with artificial colloids. In the future, oxygen-carrying perfluorocarbon and hemoglobin solutions will be of great interest to volume therapy, because they allow for the first time an increase in hemodynamics and lowering of blood viscosity without reducing oxygen-carrying capacity. I am delighted that leading scientists in this innovative and interesting field have agreed to participate in this book.

I would like to express my gratitude to Prof. Dr. K. Schimrigk, Professor emeritus of Neurology and Prof. Dr. E. Wenzel and Priv.-Doz. Dr. G. Pindur from the Department of Hemostaseology and Transfusion Medicine of the University of the Saarland, for their continuing, unrelenting support of our work and their inspiring thoughts, suggestions, and discussions.

J. Treib

Contents

Contributors

Prof. Dr. J. Boldt
Abteilung für Anästhesiologie und Intensivmedizin,
Klinikum der Stadt Ludwigshafen, 67063 Ludwigshafen, Germany

Prof. D. J. Cole M.D.
Department of Anesthesiology, Loma Linda University Medical Center,
Loma Linda, California, USA

Dr. F. Cortbus
Neurochirurgische Klinik,
Universitätskliniken des Saarlandes, 66421 Homburg, Germany

Dr. M. T. Grauer
Neurologische Klinik, Universitätskliniken des Saarlandes,
66421 Homburg, Germany

Prof. Dr. A. Haass
Neurologische Klinik, Universitätskliniken des Saarlandes,
66421 Homburg, Germany

Prof. Dr. H. Iro
Klinik für Hals-Nasen-Ohrenheilkunde,
Universitätskliniken des Saarlandes, 66421 Homburg, Germany

Prof. E. T. Riley M.D.
Department of Anesthesia, Stanford University School of Medicine,
Stanford, CA 94305, USA

Prof. Dr. K. W. Ruprecht
Augenklinik, Universitätskliniken des Saarlandes, 66421 Homburg,
Germany

Prof. R. Schell M.D.
Department of Anesthesiology, Loma Linda University Medical Center,
Loma Linda, California, USA

Dr. V. Scherer
Augenklinik, Universitätskliniken des Saarlandes, 66421 Homburg,
Germany

Prof. Dr. W. I. Steudel
Neurochirurgische Klinik, Universitätskliniken des Saarlandes,
66421 Homburg, Germany

G. Stier M.D.
Department of Anesthesiology, Loma Linda University Medical Center,
Loma Linda, California, USA

Priv.-Doz. Dr. J. Treib
Neurologische Klinik, Universitätskliniken des Saarlandes,
66421 Homburg, Germany

Dr. F. Waldfahrer
Klinik für Hals-Nasen-Ohrenheilkunde,
Universitätskliniken des Saarlandes, 66421 Homburg, Germany

Chapter 1

Volume Therapy in Neurology

J. Treib, M. T. Grauer, A. Haass

Hemodynamics in Patients with Acute Stroke

Summary

During the acute phase of stroke, the hemodynamic situation is of decisive importance. Because of the impaired autoregulation, the perfusion of the ischemic penumbra depends directly on blood pressure and cardiac output. It is a well-known fact that blood pressure is increased in the initial phase of acute stroke. Cardiac output during the initial phase of acute stroke has only been measured in individual cases.

We measured cardiac output and blood pressure non-invasively in 30 patients with acute brain stroke that did not suffer from cardiac insufficiency and in a control group with 30 patients that was matched for age, and gender. The data was correlated with clinical parameters.

Blood pressure, cardiac output and heart frequency were significantly higher in patients suffering from acute stroke compared to the control group. The longer the elapsed time between the onset of the stroke and the measurement, the higher was cardiac output. The initial Cardiac output value computed by extrapolation of the correlation curve did not differ from the mean value of the control group. We observed the statistical tendency that the heart frequency was higher in patients with more pronounced neurological symptoms. Both groups showed a positive correlation between blood pressure and age and a negative correlation between cardiac output and age.

In this study, we were able to show for the first time that patients with acute stroke that do not suffer from cardiac insufficiency have a higher cardiac output during the initial phase of acute stroke than patients in a control group. The higher cardiac output and the correlation with the age of the stroke point to a reactive, centrally triggered increase in hemodynamics.

Introduction

The incidence of brain stroke depends strongly on age. It increases from 3/100,000 in the third and fourth decade to 300/100,000 in the eight and ninth decade of life (Bonita 1992). Between the age of 45 and 85, one in four men and one in five women suffer from a brain stroke. According to the results recently published by the MONICA project of the WHO (World Health Organization Monitoring Trends and Determinants in Cardiovascular Diseases) the incidence is twice as high in Eastern Europe compared to Western Europe (Thorvaldsen et al. 1995). The study showed a decreasing incidence and prevalence during the last years, however mortality remains at an average of 30% during the first four weeks. Brain stroke remains the third-leading cause of death in industrialized countries (Bonita 1992). One third of the survivors of a brain stroke suffer from disabilities leading to a loss of independence and the necessity for nursing care. Besides the individual pain and suffering, brain stroke has a great epidemiological importance, which is bound to increase in the future as the life expectancy of the population rises.

In the industrialized nations, each year 2,000 brain strokes occur per 1 million inhabitants and 7,000 individuals per 1 million suffer from disabilities due to brain stroke. The total expenses per 1 million inhabitants are estimated to be US $ 100 million. An effective therapy that reduces morbidity and mortality would therefore have the potential to save enormous health care costs.

In the past, many patients regarded stroke with a certain fatalism, thinking that no acute therapy was available. Medical treatment was often limited to prevention and rehabilitation, where more progress was visible. The rate of re-infarction was lowered significantly through the use of platelet-aggregation inhibitors or anticoagulants (Second International Study of Infarct Survival 1988, Gent et al. 1989, Janzon et al. 1990, Marmot and Poulter 1992, European Atrial Fibrillation Trial Study Group 1993, Treib et al. 1999). Two large, prospective, randomized multi-center trials showed that for patients with symptomatic stenosis of the carotid artery, prophylactic carotid endarterectomy is superior to prevention with drugs alone (North American Symptomatic Carotid Endarterectomy Trial 1991, European Carotid Surgery Trial 1991). In patients with a symptomatic high-degree (>70%) stenosis who suffered from a transient ischemic attack in the preceding 6 months or who suffered a light brain stroke with a remission of clinical symptoms, the risk of surgery is offset by the reduced risk of brain stroke on average already after one year.

Through the creation of specialized wards for brain stroke, so called "stroke units", acute therapy was greatly improved. Langhorn et al. (1993) analyzed 10 randomized studies that were conducted between 1962 and 1993. The analysis showed that the mortality of brain stroke can be reduced by 28% compared to a normal ward, if therapy is carried out in a stroke unit. The significant difference in mortality was maintained 12 months after the onset of the stroke. The lowering of mortality did not lead to an increase in morbidity (Indredavik et al. 1991, Langhorne et al. 1993 and 1995).

The acute therapy of stroke will be improved in the future through new therapy concepts. After an analysis of the sub-groups a large, randomized double-blind study suggested that an early (<8 hours) and high-dose (12 g/day) administration of piracetam is effective in the treatment of brain stroke (De Deyn 1995). Although 3-month mortality was not reduced (22.6% with piracetam compared to 23.5% with placebo), the neurological Orgogozo-score and the Barthel-index were significantly (p<0.05) better after 4 weeks in the verum group compared to the placebo group.

Another important step in the therapy of brain stroke are the recently published results of an American multi-center study, which confirmed clinically the existence of a therapeutic window (National Institute of Neurological Disorders and Stroke rt-PA Stroke Study Group 1995). A thrombolytic therapy with a one-hour intravenous administration of 0.9 mg/kg bw recombinant tissue plasminogen activator (rt-PA) was shown to be efficacious, if therapy was initiated within three hours after the onset of symptoms. Contrary to this protocol, a comparable European multi-center study which allowed inclusion into the study up to six hours after onset of symptoms was not able to show the efficacy of the therapy (European Cooperative Acute Stroke Study 1995). The worse outcome compared to the American study was explained through the later inclusion of patients and frequently not recognized early signs of infarction, leading to increased hemorrhages into the ischemic brain region, which in turn resulted in a less favorable clinical outcome (von Kummer et al. 1995, Heiß 1996).

The piracetam study and the American rt-PA study have in common, that both therapies had no significant effect on mortality and a score improvement only after 4 weeks. Del Zoppo (1995) suspects that the test scores used to judge neurological outcomes and improvements are not sensitive enough to detect early improvements.

The American study showed that the benefit of an early thrombolysis is independent of the type of infarction. One explanation would be that reinstatement of blood flow to the ischemic region is equally important for lacunar infarctions as it is in infarctions due to occlusions of large vessels (del Zoppo 1995).

Today, therapeutic nihilism and inactivity are not justifiable anymore in acute stroke (Heiß 1996). Because effective therapy is only possible in the first few hours, it is imperative to increase awareness in the general population and in medical personnel that brain stroke is an emergency that requires immediate medical attention.

The securement of cerebral perfusion through stabilization of hemodynamics on a high level is an acknowledged goal of therapy (Heiß 1986), because a deterioration of hemodynamics through a lowering of blood pressure in the acute phase can lead to a worsening of clinical symptoms (Broderick et al. 1993, Lisk et al. 1993). Even a moderate lowering of significantly increased blood pressure is associated with the risk of increased neurological deficits (Treib et al. 1996, Fig. 1). Therefore, blood pressures that are mildly to moderately increased should not be lowered. Excessively increased blood pressures (>230/120 mm Hg) should be lowered carefully and well-controlled in the acute phase of stroke.

The results of a randomized, double-blind, placebo-controlled multi-center nimodipin study confirmed the unfavorable outcome of lowering blood pressure (Kaste et al. 1994). During the first three months, mortality in the group treated with Nimodipin (120 mg/day) was higher than in the placebo group. This was explained by the fact that nimodipin lowered systolic ($p<0.005$) and diastolic ($p<0.013$) blood pressure significantly during the first week of therapy.

From a pathophysiological perspective, blood pressure and cardiac output (CO) are of central importance in acute stroke, because ischemia tolerance of nerve tissue depends strongly on cerebral blood flow. A cerebral blood flow of 8-23 ml/100 g/min leads to a reduction in the function of nerve cells, but the viability of the cells can be maintained at least temporarily (Olsen 1986). At a cerebral blood flow of 8-16 ml/100 g/min, a complete loss of nerve cell function occurs, resulting in cell death within 1-3 hours.

The role of hemodynamics and CO for cerebral perfusion during ischemia-impaired autoregulation is not completely understood. Already 1928 it was noted that "For the development of the science of circulation it was unfortunate that blood flow is relatively difficult to measure, but blood pressure easily. For this reason, the blood pressure manometer gained an appealing importance, although most organs do not need pressure, but blood flow" (Jarisch 1928).

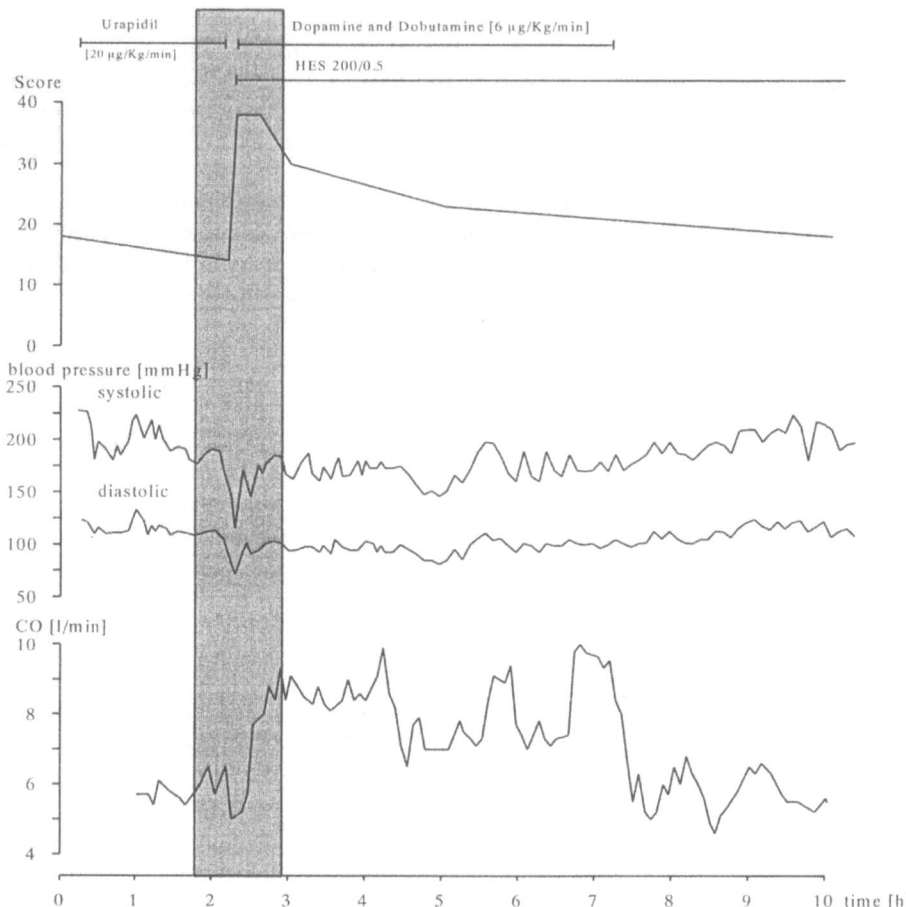

Fig. 1. Neurological score (Adams et al. 1987), systolic and diastolic pressure and cardiac output (CO) of 57-year-old patient with acute stroke. The initial blood pressure of 230/130 was lowered through i.v. administration of Urapidil. After initial improvement, clinical worsening occurred after decrease of blood pressure and CO. This decline was reversible in part through sympathomimetically supported volume therapy (modified from Treib et al. 1996)

The simplifying notion that blood pressure reflects CO is not correct, because we cannot find a correlation between these two parameters in patients with acute stroke. From clinical routine, it is well-known that a patient can have quite different CO values at equal blood pressures. With respect to cerebral blood flow the question arises, which influence blood pressure and CO in particular have on cerebral perfusion and autoregulation.

It is a well-known fact that, within the limits of physiological blood pressure, cerebral autoregulation is able to compensate a change in perfusion pressure through a change in vascular resistance and therefore to maintain through this mechanism cerebral blood flow at a constant level (Harper 1966, Powers and Raichle 1985).

The autoregulation compensates a decrease in CO only in part. Davies et al. (1980) were able to show in healthy cats that a hypovolemia-induced CO reduction of 32% results in a 24% decrease of blood flow, although blood pressure was maintained almost constant. Through administration of the beta-blocker propanolol they achieved a blood pressure-independent decrease in CO (-23%) and cerebral perfusion (-30%). However, after inducing a 72% increase in CO through hypervolemia and administration of sympathomimetics, they observed no increase in cerebral blood flow.

Werner et al. (1991) observed a blood pressure-independent decrease of cerebral blood flow after a decrease in CO although autoregulation was intact. Through administration of sufentanil to two groups of 5 dogs each, they achieved a 40-50% decline in CO. In one group, mean blood pressure decreased by 31.6%, in the other group, blood pressure was maintained constant with phenylephrine. Cerebral blood flow and flow velocity measured by transcranial doppler decreased significantly in both groups by 35-40%.

Keller et al. (1982) were able to show in primates, that local cerebral blood flow in ischemia-impaired autoregulation can be increased through raising CO. After occluding the middle cerebral artery and maintaining constant blood pressure, they achieved an increase of CO by 100-200% through a hypervolemic infusion of Dextran 40. The ischemic brain region showed subsequently a significant increase in regional cerebral blood flow, which was not observed in the non-ischemic regions. In a control group, they achieved through an isovolemic hemodilution an identical decline in hematocrit of -15%. This treatment had no significant effect on CO and blood pressure, and regional blood flow in ischemic brain regions also remained constant. The authors concluded from their experiments that the increase in cerebral blood flow after administration of volume is the result of raised CO and associated with reduced blood viscosity.

Tranmer et al. (1992) also demonstrated that it is possible to increase cerebral blood flow in ischemic brain regions by increasing CO. After unilateral occlusion of the middle cerebral artery, Tranmer et al. increased the CO of primates through infusion of starch solution by 159% and subsequently lowered CO through bloodletting to the initial level. Local cerebral blood flow correlated closely with CO (r=0.89) in the ischemic brain region, whereas blood flow in the non-ischemic region remained constant. Significant changes of blood pressure, pulse or cerebral pressure did not occur during this experiment.

Contrary to Tranmer et al., Bouma and Muizelaar (1990) were unable to detect a correlation of cerebral blood flow with CO in patients with severe head trauma and impaired autoregulation. This could be explained by the fact that the impairment of the brain tissue was traumatic and not ischemic, and that the changes in CO of the patients examined by Bouma and Muizelaar were much smaller than the changes in the primates studied by Tranmer et al.

The prognostic and therapeutic importance of CO during acute stroke is underlined through animal and human studies demonstrating that an increase of CO and blood pressure can result in a reduction of neurological deficits (Vander Ark and Pommerantz 1973, Ohtaki and Tranmer 1993).

Possibly CO is a relevant risk-factor for cerebro-vascular perfusion disorders. In cerebrovascularly healthy subjects we were able to show in a study of the circadian hemodynamic rhythm a decline of CO and pulse during the night and in the early morning (Fig. 2).

CO [l/min]

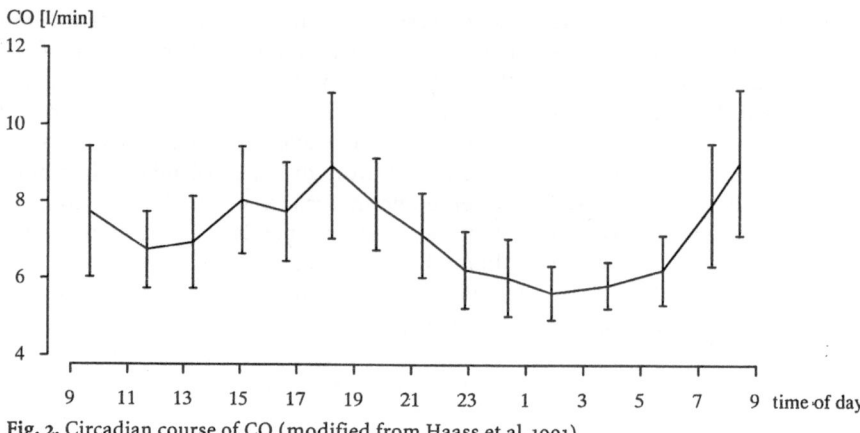

Fig. 2. Circadian course of CO (modified from Haass et al. 1991)

This decrease coincided with a drop in blood pressure observed by Millar-Craig et al. (1978) and an increase in hematocrit observed by Seaman et al. (1965). This unfavorable hemodynamic and rheologic situation, in part due to insufficient fluid intake during the night hours, explains the increased occurrence of strokes in the early morning.

Dehydration is frequent in older patients. In an American study from 1991, 6.7% of all patients admitted to a hospital were diagnosed with dehydration (Warren et al. 1994). The diagnosis can be particularly difficult in older patients, because characteristic clinical symptoms can be missing (Weinberg et al. 1995). According to a study by Bonelli and Jancusk (1984), laboratory parameters can be unreliable, because serum creatinine was increased in only 57% and hematocrit in only 28% of patients with exsiccosis that needed treatment. Measuring blood pressure can also be misleading.

A decrease in extra-cellular fluid volume leads via a reduced effective arterial blood volume to a decrease in cardiac preload and subsequently to a decline in CO and blood pressure. On the other hand, centralization and reactive increase of the sympathetic tonus together with the release of catecholamines increase peripheral vascular resistance and blood pressure (Brunner 1993). Bonelli and Jancusk (1984) therefore hold the opinion that the only reliable parameter to determine dehydration is central venous pressure. A less pronounced feeling of thirst and reduced ability of the kidneys to concentrate fluids are the main causes of the often encountered dehydration in older patients (Phillips et al. 1984, Phillips et al. 1993).

Dehydration is not only a hemodynamic and rheological risk-factor (Haaß et al. 1991), but is according to the studies by Yasaka et al. (1993) also associated with a higher rate of embolic re-infarctions. Therefore, dehydration and hypovolemia, which are often encountered in acute stroke should be treated consistently with volume therapy (Gabler-Sandberger 1996).

According to recent studies, the share of so-called hemodynamic brain strokes is about 10% (Bladin and Chambers 1994). The authors classified a stroke as hemodynamic, if the cranial CT showed a border-region infarction or so-called watershed infarctions or when patient history or clinical signs pointed to a drop in blood pressure at the time of the stroke. This is only a rough estimate, because it is seldom possible to record blood pressure and CO at the time of infarction. Another confounding factor is the increase of blood pressure after a stroke and the subsequent spontaneous drop during the course of several days after the stroke. This means that the blood pressure at the time of admittance to the hospital can be increased or already normal again (Britton and Carlsson 1986 and 1990, Broderick et al. 1993).

The etiology of the blood pressure increase after stroke is unclear. Carlberg et al. (1991) observed no correlation between the age of the infarction (time elapsed between onset of stroke and examination) and blood pressure. They suspected that mental stress during hospital admission plays a decisive role. But the early increase of blood pressure in stroke patients can with equal likelihood be attributed to an endogenous, compensatory up-regulation (Broderick et al. 1993). Smith et al. (1986) described a release of catecholamines as the cause for the increase in blood pressure. Such an up-regulation would have a positive effect on the course of the stroke, because Jörgensen et al. (1994) showed that high initial blood pressure can prevent the progression of a stroke, whereas lowering blood pressure down to normal values worsens the clinical course of the stroke (Lavin 1986, Hankey and Gubbay 1987). Also, positron emission tomography (PET) studies in hypertensive patients with cerebral perfusion disorders showed a pronounced dependency of regional cerebral blood flow on blood pressure, such that even a small decline in blood pressure can worsen cerebral perfusion (Fujii et al. 1990). For this reason, a rapid lowering of blood pressure during acute stroke is not advisable (Lavin 1986, Broderick et al. 1993, Lisk et al. 1993).

For CO, another hemodynamic parameter, only little data is available for the acute situation. Because of the equipment-intensive and invasive study methods, relevant measurements have only been carried out in individual cases. Our work attempted to close this gap through the use of the bioimpedance method.

Patients and Methods

After obtaining informed consent, we studied hemodynamics in 30 stroke patients, that were consecutively admitted to our hospital. The patients (8 women, 22 men) were not heart-insufficient and suffered from an ischemic infarction in the region of the middle cerebral artery that was less than 24 hours old.

The severity of the stroke was classified with a neurological scale (Adams et al. 1987). The control group included 30 gender- and age-matched patients without cardiovascular disorders that suffered from a non-cerebrovascular neurological disorder. In addition, we studied 7 patients with heart insufficiency and absolute arrhythmia that suffered from acute stroke.

The cardiodynamic data cardiac output (CO), heart rate and stroke volume were recorded using the bioimpedance method (NCCOM3, BoMed, Irvine, CA, USA). The bioimpedance method computes cardiodynamic parameters through the analysis of changes in impedance, i.e. changes in the resistance of alternating currents between systole and diastole (Bernstein 1986). For the measurements, a high-frequency alternating current of flow volume is applied between upper and lower thoracic aperture. The resulting changes in impedance are measured using 4 pairs of electrodes that are attached at the right and left neck and the middle axilla line at the height of the xiphoid bone. In the thorax region, blood has the lowest electrical resistance and changes in blood flow caused by the heart result in rhythmic changes of impedance. From these pulse-dependent changes in impedance, it is possible to compute CO, heart rate, stroke volume, peak flow, ejection fraction, end-diastolic volume, contractility index, acceleration index, ventricular ejection time, ejection ratio and systolic time ratio (Castor et al. 1989).

In comparison with the thermodilution method, the measurements of CO showed a good to very good correlation (r=0.88 to 0.95) (Bernstein 1986, Mattar et al. 1986, Introna et al. 1988, Castor et al. 1990, Clancy et al. 1991). The comparison with doppler-sonographic measurements also showed a good correlation (Castor et al. 1994). When measuring critically patients, the correlation coefficient dropped to r=0.56-0.86 (Appel et al. 1986, Shoemaker et al. 1988, Castor et al. 1988). During intraoperative CO measurements and in studies of respirated patients, several researchers noted an insufficient correlation between the thoracic bioimpedance and thermodilution method (Weber et al. 1986, Sommoggy et al. 1988, Castor 1994). Other sources of error are unusual shape of the thorax, inaccurate positioning of fixation of the electrodes, pronounced arrhythmia and valvular heart disease (Woo et al. 1991). Particularly in patients with aortic insufficiency the displayed values of CO are too high, because the diastolic regurgitation is not taken into account.

Regarding the accuracy of the other data computed by NCCOM3 little data is available in the literature. Except for heart frequency, which unsurprisingly shows agreement with the EKG, only studies about ejection fraction and thoracic fluid index are available. According to these studies, the displayed absolute values are correct only within limits, whereas relative, intra-individual changes are measured accurately during repeated measurements (Goldstein et al. 1986, Boldt et al. 1988, Sommoggy et al. 1988, Castor et al. 1989). Decisive advantages of the thoracic bioimpedance method are its non-invasiveness and possibility of continuous, stroke-by-stroke measurements.

Blood pressures were measured with an automatic measuring device (Sirecust 401, Siemens, Erlangen, Germany).

The data was recorded and analyzed using special software (Stoll et al. 1992). Mean value and standard deviation were computed. For non-normal samples, the median was determined. The Mann-Whitney test was used to test for significant differences between both groups. In addition, the Spearman-rank correlation coefficient and 95% confidence intervals were computed (Altman 1991). For the main parameter CO, multiple regression was carried out.

Results

Compared to the control group of cerebrovascularly healthy subjects, the CO values of the stroke patients were significantly ($p<0.01$) increased by 14.5% on admission to the hospital (Table 1).

We observed the statistical tendency that the CO was higher, when the elapsed time between the stroke and the measurements was longer (r=0.33, p=0.07 [-0.04; 0.61] Fig. 3). Through extrapolation of the correlation curve, a CO value at the time of the onset of the stroke was computed. This CO value did not differ from the mean

Table 1. Clinical and hemodynamic data of 30 patients with acute stroke and a control group (modified from Treib et al. 1996)

	Acute stroke	Control group	Significance
Age of patients	62.4±10.5	62.6±14.7	n. s.
Systolic blood pressure (mmHg)	152.8±21.3	142.1±17.4	$p<0.05$
Diastolic blood pressure (mmHg)	91.6±9.8	86.2±9.7	$p<0.05$
Cardiac output (l/min)	6.3±1.5	5.5±20.0	$P<0.01$
Heart rate (l/min)	84.7±17.3	76.4±12.5	$p<0.05$
Stroke volume (ml)	73.3±25.1	73.5±28.0	n. s.
Severity of stroke (Adam's Score)	40.5±25.2	—	
Time after onset of stroke (h)	8.3±6.1	—	

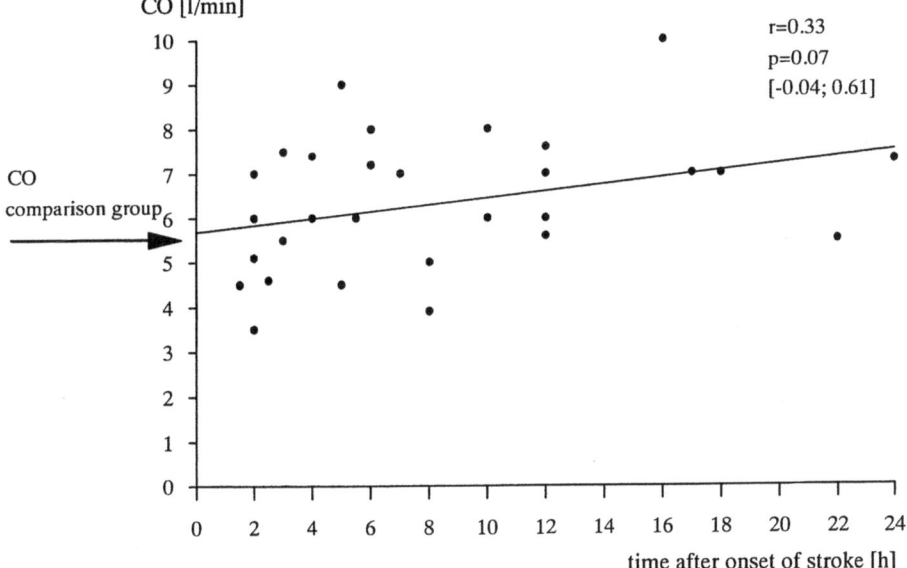

Fig. 3. Dependence of CO on age of stroke, measured in 30 patients without cardiac insufficiency with acute stroke on time of admission to the hospital. The arrow marks the average CO of a control group, matched for age and gender, without cerebrovascular problems (modified from Treib et al. 1996)

value of the control group (5.6 vs. 5.5 l/min). CO decreased significantly with the age of the stroke patients (r=-0.37, p<0.05 [-0.64; -0.01] Fig. 4) and the control group (r=-0.53, p<0.01 [-0.74; -0.2]). Both groups showed a significant correlation between CO and stroke volume (r=0.61, p<0.01 [0.32; 0.79] vs. r=0.83, p<0.01 [0.66; 0.91]).

In a multiple regression model, a significant regression coefficient was obtained for CO and age of infarction, adjusted for patient age (CO = 10.35+0.094 x age of infarction - 0.077 x age of patient). The confidence interval for the age of infarction was [0.018; 0.170] at p=0.017. For patient age, a confidence interval of [-0.121; -0.033] at p=0.001 was computed. Systolic and diastolic blood pressure as well as the severity of the stroke had no significant effect on CO in the multiple regression model.

blood pressure [mmHg]

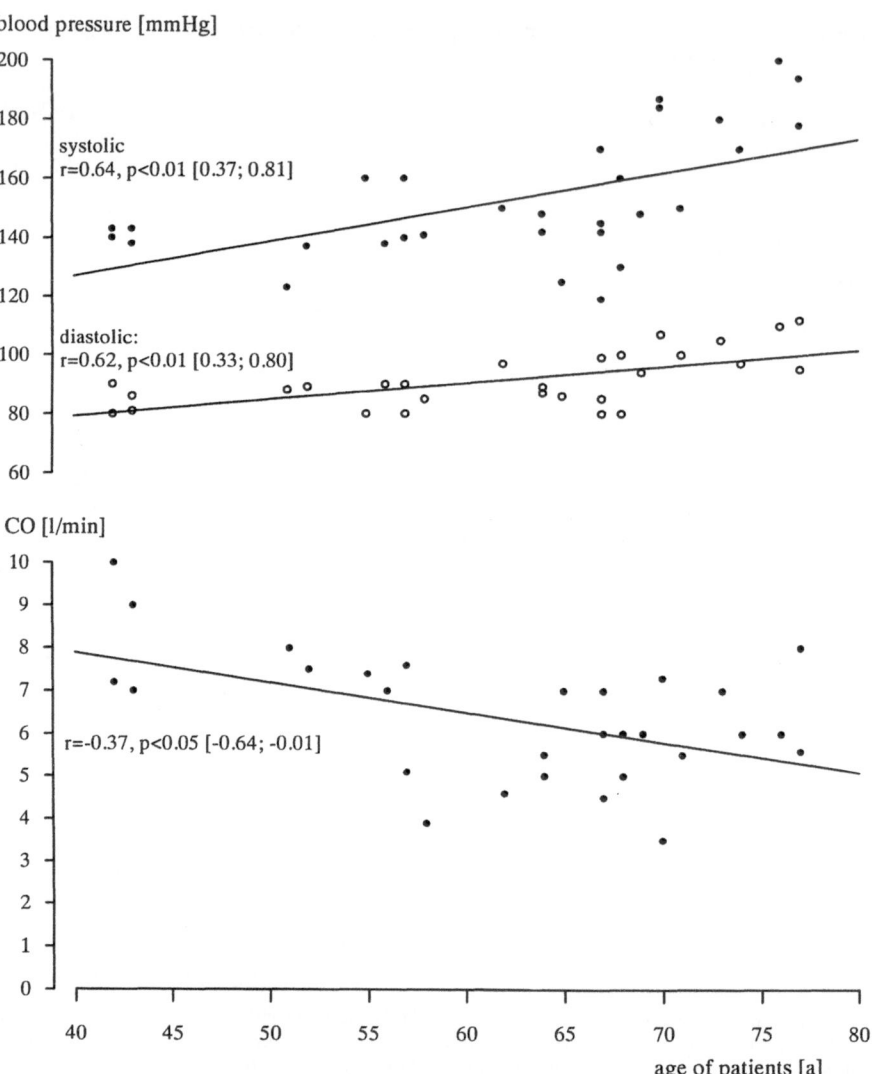

Fig. 4. Dependence of CO and blood pressure on age, measured in 30 acute stroke patients without cardiac insufficiency on time of admission (modified from Treib et al. 1996)

The mean time between the onset of symptoms and the clinical examination was 8.3 hours. There was no significant correlation between earlier arrival in the clinic and the severity of neurological deficits (r=-0.27, p=0.15 [-0.57; 0.10].

In the stroke patient group, systolic and diastolic blood pressure increased with age (r=0.64, p<0.01 vs. r=0.62, p<0.01). The stroke patients had significantly higher systolic and diastolic blood pressures on admission to the hospital. There was no significant correlation between systolic and diastolic blood pressures and the time

Table 2. Clinical and hemodynamic data of patients with acute stroke suttering from absolute arrhythmia

	Acute stroke
Age of patients	74.0±9.0
Systolic blood pressure (mmHg)	161.2±17.5
Diastolic blood pressure (mmHg)	91.2±7.8
Cardiac output (l/min)	3.6±0.5
Heart rate (l/min)	96.0±14.9
Stroke volume (ml)	36.4±7.4
Severity of stroke (Adam's Score)	57.0±20.6
Time after onset of stroke (h)	4.1±1.8

elapsed between the onset of the infarction and the measurement of the blood pressure ($r=0.04$ vs. $r=0.07$).

We observed a statistically not significant trend that heart frequency was higher in patients with more severe neurological deficits ($r=0.28$; $p=0.11$ [-0.09; 0.58]). In stroke patients, the decrease in stroke volume correlated significantly with heart frequency ($r=-0.41$; $p<0.05$). This correlation was not observed in the control group ($r=-0.3$, n.s.).

Seven additional patients with acute stroke suffered from absolute arrhythmia (Table 2). Neurological deficits in this patient group were more severe and time elapsed between the onset of symptoms and admission to the hospital was shorter (4.1 vs. 8.3 hours). These patients were on average 12 years older. Systolic blood pressure and pulse of these patients were 8.4 mmHg and 11.3/s higher, respectively. CO and stroke volume were 2.7 l/min and 36.9 ml lower, respectively, than in stroke patients without heart insufficiency. Compared to the control group, systolic blood pressure and heart frequency of the stroke patients with absolute arrhythmia were 19.1 mmHg and 19.6/s higher, respectively. CO and stroke volume were 1.9 l/min and 37.1 ml lower, respectively, than in the control group of patients that were cerebrovascularly healthy.

Discussion

This study showed that patients with acute stroke have a significantly higher CO than a control group that has been matched for age, gender and cardiac parameters. The higher CO and the significant regression between CO and age of infarction suggest that CO increases during the first hours of an acute stroke (Treib et al. 1996). The reactive, probably centrally triggered increase of hemodynamics is possibly caused by a release of catecholamines (Smith et al. 1986, Hamann 1993, Sander and Klingelhöfer 1994).

In agreement with earlier studies, patients with acute stroke had a significantly higher initial blood pressure than a comparable control group (Britton and Carlsson 1986 and 1990, Carlberg et al. 1991, Broderick et al. 1993). Again, no correlation between blood pressure and age of infarction was found. The significantly higher initial blood pressures at time of the onset of the stroke can be explained through a reactive, centrally triggered increase blood pressure or a higher percentage of hypertensive patients among the stroke patients. Since blood pressure drops spontaneously in the first few days after the stroke (Britton and Carlsson 1986 and 1990, Carlberg et al. 1991, Broderick et al. 1993), the significantly higher initial blood pressure can only be explained in part with a higher share of hypertensive patients.

The etiologic inhomogeneity of strokes complicates the analysis and interpretation of hemodynamic studies considerably. Hemodynamics has a different relevance for an embolic occlusion of the middle cerebral artery than for a hemodynamic or lacunar infarction (Ringelstein et al. 1989 and 1990). A hemodynamic stroke is caused by a worsening of hemodynamics and results in the formation of so-called watershed or border-zone infarctions. In the case of an embolic infarction of the middle cerebral artery, caused for example by a cardiac embolic source, hemodynamics plays a lesser role in the pathogenesis of the infarction. Sander and Klingelhöfer (1994) were able to show that both types of infarctions because of their differing localization and area of expansion and also because of differing norepinephrine concentrations lead to different circadian blood pressure patterns. According to this study, the involvement of the insula cortex plays an important role. The effects of lacunar infarctions were not described by the authors. Due to the smaller area of expansion, hemodynamic effects of lacunar infarctions are probably smaller.

Also, hemodynamic effects of a stroke depend on the cardiac health of the patient. The study results of Staedt (1994) suggest that patients with cardiac insufficiency show little or no increase in CO. Contrary to our study, Staedt observed in patients with acute stroke a significantly lower CO and stroke volume compared to a cardiovascularly healthy control group. One possible explanation could be that 41% of the stroke patients in Staedt's study suffered from myocardial insufficiency, whereas this was an exclusion criterion in our study.

The view that patients with cardiac insufficiency should be regarded separately with respect to hemodynamics is supported by the results of our study with 7 patients who suffered from cardiac insufficiency and absolute arrhythmia. This patient group was 12 years older on average and their neurological scores were 41% lower compared to other stroke patients. Systolic blood pressure and pulse were 5.4% and 13.3% higher, respectively, CO and stroke volume were 42.8% and 50.3% lower, respectively. One has to consider however, that for CO and stroke volume, the bioimpedance method loses accuracy in patients with cardiac arrhythmias.

From a pathophysiological perspective, the severe neurological deficits of the patients with absolute arrhythmia could be the result of a larger, embolus-induced infarction of the region perfused by the middle cerebral artery, presumably caused by a cardiac emboly source. Another reason for the severe deficits could be an insufficient collateral supply of the penumbra due to limited cardiac competence and subsequently lower CO.

Influence of an Iso- and Hypervolemic Volume Therapy on Hemodynamics in Patients with Acute Stroke

Summary

Past clinical hemodilution studies have yielded conflicting results. Whereas isovolemic therapy studies showed no clinical improvement, hypervolemic volume therapies suggested clinical benefits. This was explained by an improvement of rheological parameters and CO through hypervolemic hemodilution in patients with sufficient cardiac competence. Up to this point, clinical studies were missing.

We measured the hemodynamic effects of isovolemic and hypervolemic hemodilution therapy using the thoracic bioimpedance method. Isovolemic hemodilution did not result in an increase of CO and blood pressure. Hypervolemic hemodilution in patients with cardiac competence increased CO by about 15%. However, this increase lasted only 3 hours. In patients with cardiac insufficiency, a slow increase in CO could only be observed after the administration of digitalis.

In patients with cardiac insufficiency, hypervolemic hemodilution alone did not achieve a sufficient increase in CO. Therefore, volume therapy should be adjusted individually to the cardiac competence of the hydration state of the patient.

Introduction

Hemodilution therapy is a frequently used therapy for cerebral perfusion disorders. The concept is based on the measurements of regional cerebral blood flow published by von Gottstein (1965). The measurements showed an increase of regional cerebral blood flow in patients with anemia and a decrease in patients with polycythemia. An increase of brain perfusion after therapeutic lowering of the hematocrit has been shown repeatedly (Gottstein and Held 1969, Thomas et al. 1977 and 1982, Gottstein 1986, Hino et al. 1994). When autoregulation is intact, this increase in brain perfusion is based on compensatory vasodilation due to reduced oxygen carrying capacity of the blood.

In ischemia-induced impairment of cerebral autoregulation, decreased as well as increased hematocrit levels lead to a worsening of hypoxia. Kiyohara et al. (1985) were able to show in studies with rats that lactate and adenosine triphosphate concentrations as well as the lactate/pyruvate quotient show a u-shaped correlation with hematocrit in the ischemic brain. The optimal value was a hematocrit of 37%. In non-ischemic control rats, they observed no dependency of brain metabolite concentrations on hematocrit levels.

This study is supported by the work of Yamauchi et al. (1993). Using positron emission tomography (PET), this group was able to show in patients with cerebral perfusion disorders caused by an occlusion of the internal carotid artery that an isovolemic lowering of hematocrit from 41.2% to 36.3% results in an increase of cerebral blood flow and oxygen transport in the ischemic brain region.

The fact that hematocrit is a risk-factor for the incidence and prognosis of brain stroke is another supporting argument for therapeutic lowering of the hematocrit. In a 16-year long prospective study, Kiyohara et al. (1986) observed that a decreased as well as an increased hematocrit are risk-factors for cerebral perfusion disorders. According to this study, the optimal hematocrit levels are below 35% for men and 30-40% for women. Wannamethee et al. (1994) showed that an increased hematocrit (>51%) is an independent risk factor, acting synergistically with increased blood pressure.

Furthermore, after analyzing cranial CTs, Harrison et al. (1981) found a correlation between the size of an infarction and the level of hematocrit. Lowe et al. (1983) showed the higher hematocrit at the time of admission to the hospital, the higher stroke mortality. Perez-Trepichio et al. (1992) confirmed this in a rat model. After triggering embolic strokes, they lowered hematocrit from 46% to 35% within 30 minutes through an isovolemic hemodilution with hydroxyethylstarch (HES) 200/0.5 and achieved a significant (p<0.05) reduction of infarction volume by 89% when compared to the control group.

The data in the literature concerning the optimal hematocrit for a hemodilution therapy ranges from 33% to 42%, with a tendency to values between 37% and 42% during the last years (Kusunoki et al. 1981, Thomas et al. 1982, Wood et al. 1982, Grossman 1983, Kiesewetter et al. 1987, Haaß et al. 1991 and 1994, Marx et al. 1995). However, "optimal" hematocrit certainly is no fixed value. Rather, it depends on individual hemodynamic and rheological parameters and the vascular status of the patient. Also, animal data cannot be directly transferred to humans. Therefore, the "optimal" hematocrit range in an older patient with arteriosclerotic vessels and limited cardiac competence will probably be higher than in a healthy animal, which can compensate a decrease in oxygen carrying capacity much better through an increase in circulatory output (Haaß et al. 1991).

In addition, in-vitro studies are of limited value. Pries and Gaehtgens were able to show that the results of glass capillary measurements reflect the complex environment of a microcirculatory, mesenteric network only insufficiently (Pries et al. 1990, 1992, 1994 and 1995). The authors observed in a mesenteric microcirculatory network a higher flow resistance than in comparable glass capillaries, which they attributed to the complex interactions of blood components with vascular endothelium that do not occur in glass capillaries (Pries et al. 1994). Furthermore, most in-vitro studies do not take into account the pulsatile blood flow in-vivo. Compared to a quantitatively comparable, non-pulsatile blood flow, a pulsatile blood flow in ischemic regions results in a greater local blood flow, a phenomenon which has not been explained satisfactorily (Tranmer et al. 1986).

One also has to bear in mind that hematocrit in the microcirculation is considerably lower than in the macro-circulation, due to the Fåhraeus-Lindqvist- and erythrocyte-sieve effect. Koscielny et al. (1991) observed in a microscopic capillary study of skin capillaries that the decrease in capillary hematocrit (-8.2%) through isovolemic hemodilution is only half as large as the decrease of hematocrit in the macro-circulation (-17.9%). On the other hand, a hypervolemic hemodilution resulted in no significant decrease in capillary hematocrit, so that oxygen carrying capacity at constant oxygen content increased significantly due to accelerated blood flow.

Lin et al. (1995) confirmed these observations for the microcirculation in animal experiments. An isovolemic hemodilution lowered systemic hematocrit by 38%, compared to the control group, however the drop in hematocrit in the microcirculation was considerably lower (13%). In the hemodilution group, oxygen release was 9% higher and local cerebral blood flow 59% higher than in the control group. At the same time, erythrocyte transit time was shorter (-15%).

The search for an "optimal" hematocrit should not focus exclusively on optimal oxygen release, because the plasma-mediated transport of metabolites is of decisive importance in ischemia-impaired microcirculation. According to animal studies carried out by Lin et al. (1995), a significant reduction of plasma transit time (-46%) can be achieved in the cerebral microcirculation through hemodilution therapy.

Another positive effect of hemodilution consists of homogenizing erythrocyte flow between the proximal and distal vascular network regions (Pries et al. 1992). A further possible mechanism of hemodilution therapy is the lowering of post-ischemic leukocyte adhesion mediated through a coating effect of colloidal plasma substitutes. However, current data on this is contradictory and does not allow any final conclusions (Menger 1995).

Hemodilution can be carried out in two ways: isovolemic, through bloodletting and substitution of the same volume through plasma expanders or hypervolemic through infusion of plasma substitutes with no or little bloodletting. Isovolemic hemodilution results in a greater lowering of hematocrit and offers the advantage of reduced cardiac burden. In patients with sufficient cardiac competence, hypervolemic therapy has the advantage of increasing CO.

The concept of isovolemic hemodilution during acute stroke with the exclusive goal of lowering blood viscosity has been shown to be ineffective in clinical studies so far (Scandinavian Stroke Study Group 1987 and 1988, Italian Acute Stroke Study Group 1988, Mast and Marx 1991 and 1992). Subsequently, the whole concept of hemodilution was questioned (Back and von Kummer 1989, Adams et al. 1994). The negative result of these studies was explained by the proponents of hemodilution therapy through methodological problems, the use of the rheologically unfavorable plasma substitute Dextran 40 and by the fact that hematocrit was lowered in some cases below 35% which is a consequence of animal studies, whose results cannot be directly applied to humans. In addition it was suspected that, contrary to hypervolemic hemodilution, an isovolemic hemodilution leads to no hemodynamic improvement (Haaß et al. 1991, Marx et al. 1995).

Hypervolemic hemodilution therapy attempts not only to optimize hematocrit, but also to improve cerebral perfusion through an increase in CO (Wood et al. 1982 and 1983, Grotta et al. 1985 and 1987). The results of an American multi-center study (Hemodilution in Stroke Study Group 1989) and the studies by Strand et al. (1984), Koller et al. (1990), Haaß et al. (1991), Goslinga et al. (1992) and Aichner et al. (1998) support within limits the effectiveness of this concept. A sub-group analysis of the American study showed that hypervolemic hemodilution reduces neurological deficits of stroke patients better than the standard therapy, if the treatment begins within 12 hours, hematocrit is lowered by 15% and CO is raised by at least 10%.

Strand et al. (1992) observed in a follow-up study that hemodilution-induced improvement of the patients treated on his specialized ward was upheld one year after therapy. The number of survivors in the hemodilution group was not significantly higher than in the control group (36 vs. 30), but the neurological deficits of hemodiluted patients were significantly ($p<0.05$) lower. The share of severely disabled patients in the hemodilution group was 6%, in the control group it was 30%. The share of patients that were able to walk was also significantly higher (92% vs. 73%).

The clinical hemodilution studies carried out so far suggest that a lowering of the hematocrit only leads to clinical improvement, when it is accompanied by an increase in CO. However, studies concerning the effect of isovolemic and hypervolemic hemodilution on hemodynamics have not yet been conducted.

Patients and Methods

Isovolemic Hemodilution

An isovolemic therapy according to the protocol of the Italian multi-center study was carried out (Italian Acute Stroke Study Group 1988). 6 Patients without cardiac insufficiency that suffered from chronic cerebrovascular perfusion disorders underwent bloodletting and infusion of Dextran 40.

Hypervolemic Hemodilution in Patients without Cardiac Insufficiency

In a second group, 6 patients without cardiac insufficiency and chronic cerebro-vascular perfusion disorders underwent hypervolemic hemodilution. The treatment consisted of the administration of a loading dose of 500 ml 10% HES 200/0.5 and 500 ml electrolyte solution. Therapy was then continued with a long-term infusion of 1000 ml HES and 1000 ml electrolyte solution over 24 hours.

Hypervolemic Hemodilution in Patients with Cardiac Insufficiency

This group consisted of 6 patients with cardiac insufficiency (NYHA II-III) who had an infarction in the region of the middle cerebral artery that was up to 24 hours old. The patients underwent hypervolemic hemodilution and received a loading dose of 500 ml 10% HES 200/0.5 and electrolyte solution, followed by a long-term infusion of a maximum of 1000 ml HES and 1000 ml electrolyte solution. The central venous pressure was monitored. At the same time, heeding contraindications, patients received three times 0.2 mg digoxin intravenously.

In all 3 groups patients with a fresh myocardial infarction, manifest coronary heart disease, increased extra-systoles, blood pressure over 200/110 mmHg, pulse over 120/min, coagulation disorders or renal insufficiency were excluded. Informed consent was obtained.

Blood pressure was recorded with an automatic blood pressure measuring device. Cardiodynamic data was recorded with the thoracic bioimpedance measuring device NCCOM3 (BoMed, Irvine, CA, USA).

Results

Isovolemic Hemodilution

Isovolemic hemodilution, i.e. the administration of volume after bloodletting, resulted in no increase of CO and blood pressure (Fig. 5). During bloodletting, a short drop in CO was observed. The course of CO did not differ from the circadian rhythm of untreated subjects (Fig. 2).

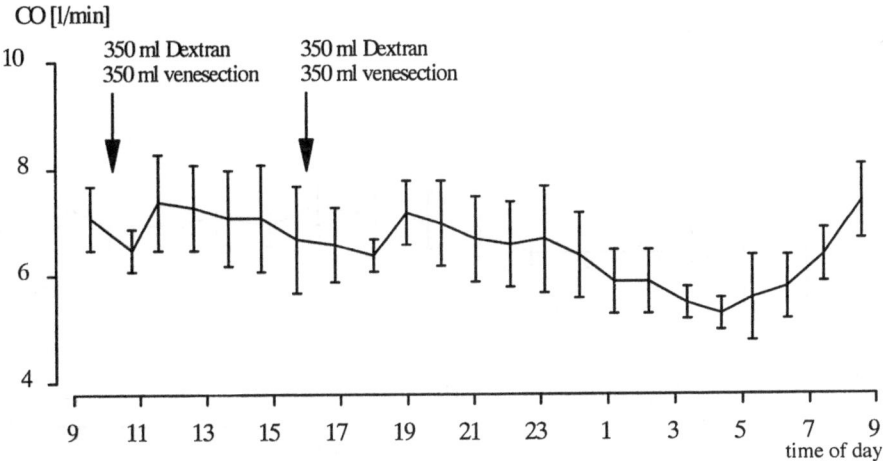

Fig. 5. Effect of isovolemic hemodilution therapy according to the protocol of the Italian Acute Stroke Study Group (1988) on CO

Hypervolemic Hemodilution in Patients without Cardiac Insufficiency

During the loading dose, a rapid, 15% increase of CO=Cardiac output that last approximately 3 hours was observed in patients without cardiac insufficiency (Fig. 6).

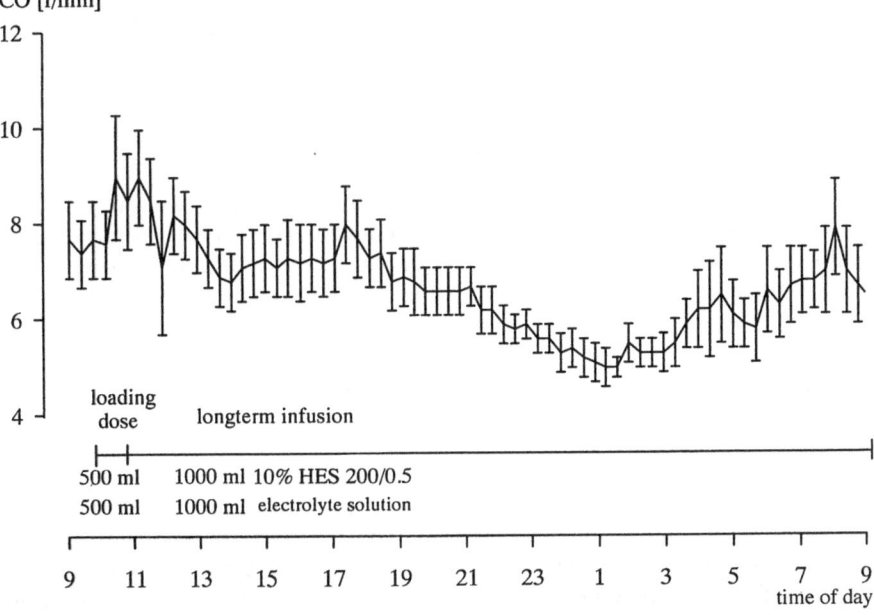

Fig. 6. Effect of hypervolemic hemodilution on CO in patient with cerebral perfusion disorders and without cardiac insufficiency (modified from Treib et al. 1996)

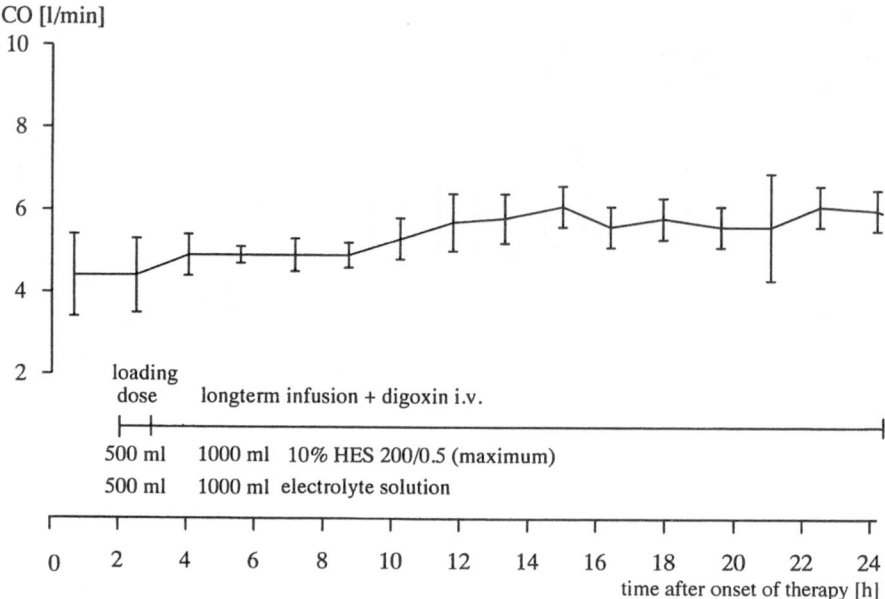

Fig. 7. Effect of a hypervolemic hemodilution with additional digoxin on the CO of patients with cardiac insufficiency and acute stroke (modified from Treib et al. 1996)

This increase in CO was mostly due to an increase in stroke volume and was not accompanied by relevant changes in pulse or blood pressure. Subsequently, CO dropped to the initial value. During the night, the patients showed a physiological decrease in CO, which can also be observed in untreated subjects (Fig. 2).

Hypervolemic Hemodilution in Patients with Cardiac Insufficiency

On admission, CO of the acute stroke patients with cardiac insufficiency was only 4.4 l/min. During the loading dose, no increase in CO was observed. During the further course of the therapy after administration of digoxin, CO increased to approximately 6 l/min (Fig. 7). Because all patients were acute cases, time of therapy onset varied. Contrary to the first two groups, hours after onset of therapy were plotted on the x-axis.

Discussion

In this study it became apparent, that patients with acute stroke are in an unfavorable hemodynamic situation, if they suffer at the same time from myocardial insufficiency. From a pathophysiological perspective, low CO and blood pressure values are unfavorable in the acute situation, because the perfusion of the ischemic penumbra depends directly on blood pressure and CO, since autoregulation is impaired. Under therapeutic aspects, it seems therefore reasonable to normalize or even raise cardiovascular parameters in the acute situation.

The hemodynamic studies showed that isovolemic hemodilution does not increase CO and blood pressure. Moreover, a too rapid bloodletting causes a short decline in CO. This lack of hemodynamic improvement together with the pronounced decline in hematocrit probably explains the clinical worsening that have been repeatedly observed under isovolemic hemodilution (Italian Stroke Study Group 1988, Mast and Marx 1991).

Due to the Frank-Starling mechanism, administration of volume improves ventricular filling and raises CO via an increase in stroke volume, an effect which has been confirmed in several studies (Wood et al. 1983, Hankeln et al. 1988). Using trans-esophageal echo-cardiographic monitoring in cardiovascularly healthy patients undergoing a preoperative hypervolemic hemodilution, van Daele et al. (1994) observed that an infusion of 1500 ml Dextran 40 and 1500 ml Ringer solution resulted in a 36% deincrease of hematocrit. The increase in CO was due to an increase in stroke volume from 48 to 72 ml, while heart frequency remained constant. The increase in wedge pressure from 5.9 to 22.6 mmHg did not lead to cardiac dilation.

The study also demonstrated that not all stroke patients profit equally from the administration of volume. In patients without cardiac insufficiency, hypervolemic hemodilution caused during the phase of the loading dose an increase in CO, which subsided after several hours, probably because of endogenous counter-regulatory mechanisms. In patients that suffered from cardiac insufficiency, the administration of volume alone did not suffice to achieve a sufficient increase in CO. On admission, the CO of these patients was 40% lower than in healthy patients and reacted towards external triggers with small changes only. Because most patients were dehydrated and had a high hematocrit, the reason for this was most likely hypovolemia. A rapid administration of volume resulted in these patients in a small or no increase of CO. A patient with cardiac insufficiency can react towards increased filling of the ventricles with only a small increase in stroke volume. Moreover, increasing cardiac preload raises stroke volume only up to a certain limit, and in patients with manifest cardiac insufficiency, preload can already be increased at rest.

Keller et al. (1982) observed comparable effects in animal experiments. After occluding the middle cerebral artery in primates, the authors carried out a volume therapy with Dextran 40 to increase CO and measured regional cerebral blood flow. In primates with cardiac insufficiency, CO rose continuously to 0.64 l/min until pulmonary artery wedge pressure reached 14 mmHg. At the same time, regional cerebral blood flow in the ischemic areas increased. After reaching a wedge pressure of 20 mmHg, CO dropped more than half to 0.31 l/min and regional cerebral blood flow dropped in the ischemic brain regions as well. When wedge pressure was decreased again, CO and regional cerebral blood flow increased to the initial value.

The lacking increase in CO in our patients was no sign of a cardiac decompensation neither by clinical or laboratory parameters, because no hemodynamic or neurological deterioration was observed under the therapy.

Administration of volume, particularly in patients with cardiac insufficiency, should never be carried out in a schematic way. It has to be adjusted individually according to fluid balance and cardiac competence. Fluid administration should be tightly monitored and limited in time. A stabilized cardiovascular situation with high-normal cardiac preload is a favorable basis for the use of inotropically positive substances. Administration of digitalis only achieves a slow increase in CO (Goldstein et al. 1980). Because of their rapid onset and the much stronger positive inotropic effect, sympathomimetics are useful to increase hemodynamics (Kulka and Tryba 1993).

Sympathomimetically Supported Volume Therapy in Patients with Acute Stroke

Summary

Hypervolemic hemodilution alone does not lead to a long-lasting increase of hemodynamics. In a pilot study, we therefore examined the effect of a combined therapy with dopamine/dobutamine and administration of volume on the cardiovascular and clinical parameters of 24 patients with an infarction of the middle cerebral artery. Using transcranial doppler sonography (TCD), the effect of blood pressure and CO on blood flow in the middle cerebral artery was studied.

From the clinical course, it was possible to divide the patients in two groups. 13 patients showed direct improvement under therapy. 11 patients showed no or delayed clinical improvement. The patients with clinical improvement showed under a stepwise increase of the dopamine/dobutamine dose a 30% increase of CO and heart frequency within one hour. Blood pressure was raised by only 10%. At the same time, the neurological score improved by 30%. In the group without neurological score improvement, the increase in hemodynamics was only half as large. In the affected brain hemisphere, flow velocity measured by TCD was significantly ($p<0.05$) lower by one-fourth compared to the unaffected side. Under therapy, systolic flow velocity rose in the unaffected hemisphere by 27%. In the affected hemisphere, flow velocity increased by only 11%, due to the impaired autoregulation. In the ischemic region, the correlation between mean flow velocity and blood pressure was more significant ($r=0.44$; $p<0.01$ [0.22; 0.62]) than the correlation between mean flow velocity and CO ($r=0.20$; $p<0.10$ [-0.04; 0.43].

This pilot study showed in the acute phase of ischemic stroke a direct correlation between an improvement of hemodynamics and an improvement of neurological scores. Unfavorable prognostic factors are higher age, limit cardiac competence and severe neurological deficits.

Introduction

The concept of increasing cardiac parameters through sympathomimetically supported volume therapy has its origins in the treatment of surgical high-risk patients (Boyd et al. 1993). Shoemaker et al. (1982) noted that survivors of high-risk operations have initially significantly higher CO values than non-survivors. In a randomized study, they showed that mortality compared to a control group can be lowered significantly from 48% to 13%. This was possible by raising CO to the mean value of survivors (cardiac index >4.5 l/min/m$_2$), whereas the target in the control group was in the normal range (cardiac index 2.8-3.5 l/min/m$_{2)}$ (Shoemaker et al. 1982, 1988 and 1993). Through such a hyperdynamic volume therapy it was also possible to lower mortality and morbidity of patients with trauma and sepsis (Flemming et al. 1992, Shoemaker et al. 1993, Bishop et al. 1993). To increase hemodynamics, dobutamine as well as colloidal and crystalloid plasma substitutes were used (Shoemaker et al. 1989, 1990).

Hyperdynamic therapy has been used in recent years to treat vasospasm in subarachnoid hemorrhage. Otsubo et al. (1990) observed under normovolemic hypertension-inducing therapy a reduction of neurological deficits in 17 of 24 patients. The authors administered dopamine and dobutamine up to a maximum dose of 20µg/kg bw and infused low-molecular weight Dextran for 7 days to compensate hypovolemia. Levy et al (1993) carried out a dobutamine-supported hypervolemic therapy in 23 patients and achieved a 52% increase in cardiac output and an 11% increase in blood pressure through the infusion of 5% albumin solution and dobutamine (5 to 10 µg/kg bw). This treatment lead to a reduction of neurological deficits in 18 of 23 patients. Mori et al. (1995) confirmed these positive clinical experiences in the treatment of vasospasm with hypervolemic hemodilution and attributed the good outcome of their patients to the significant increase in CO (+35%) and blood pressure (+12%) as well as the lowering of hematocrit and erythrocyte aggregation.

Based on these positive experiences in the treatment of vasospasm, we carried out a circulation-supporting volume therapy in patients with acute stroke. As plasma substitute, we used HES 200/0.5, which has a stable volume effect, favorable rheological and pharmacokinetic properties and does not affect coagulation negatively (Treib et al. 1995–1999). Before the administration of catecholamines, it is important to balance out hypovolemia. Because otherwise the administration of dobutamine can lead to a reduction in blood pressure, due to beta-receptor mediated lowering of peripheral resistance (Kulka and Tryba 1993).

At the moment, it is the subject of discussion whether strongly increased blood pressure levels carry the dangers of hemorrhage into the infarction, worsening of the ischemic brain edema and damage to the blood-brain barrier and up to which blood pressure levels the benefits of an improved perfusion outweigh the risks (Aspey et al. 1987, Harrison 1992, Del Zoppo 1995, Dandapani et al. 1995, Leys et al. 1995). Possibly, the correlation between blood pressure and outcome and CO and outcome is not linear, but U-shaped (Irie et al. 1993). It is universally accepted that blood pressure and CO levels below the normal range are unfavorable for the outcome, due to insufficient cerebral perfusion pressure. No scientifically validated data is available about the "optimal blood pressure" or the "optimal CO" in acute stroke. Regarding strongly increased blood pressure and CO levels, animal and clinical studies are insufficient and have yielded conflicting results.

Fenske et al. (1978) found in a cat-model after the occlusion of the middle cerebral artery signs for an increase in ischemic brain edema through arterial hypertension, whereas Yamaguchi et al. (1989) noted in a similar experimental setup signs of a suppression of brain edema in the core zone through maintenance of a high perfusion pressure. Dandapani et al. (1995) observed in a retrospective study in patients with brain hemorrhage that clearly elevated initial blood pressure levels (mean blood pressure >145 mmHg) affect the clinical course negatively. Jörgensen et al. (1994) on the other hand computed in a prospective study of 868 patients with brain stroke that a higher blood pressure reduces the danger of progression of a stroke by a factor of 0.66 per 20 mmHg.

Goal of the present study was to examine the effect of hemodynamics on the cerebral autoregulation of the affected and non-affected vascular region and to correlate this data with the clinical course. To study the effect of blood pressure and CO on cerebral autoregulation, we used transcranial doppler sonography (TCD). In the acute situation of a stroke, using TCD, it is possible to rapidly gain information about cerebral flow velocity and cerebral autoregulation without the need for expensive or cumbersome equipment. Contrary to single photon emission computer tomography (SPECT) and positron emission tomography (PET), TCD is useful for the continuous monitoring of hemodynamic therapy concepts in acute stroke. According to animal studies by Werner et al. (1991), a close correlation (r=0.82) exists between TCD flow velocity and cerebral blood flow.

Patients and Methods

To improve hemodynamics, 24 patients with an acute ischemic stroke in the region of the middle cerebral artery underwent a combination therapy, consisting of dopamine/dobutamine and administration of volume in an intensive-care setting. After obtaining informed consent, 24 patients whose infarction was less than 24 hours old and had not yet demarcated itself as hypodensity in the cranial CT, were included into the study.

Excluded were patients with hemodynamically relevant extra-cranial stenoses, manifest coronary insufficiency, myocardial infarction within the last four weeks, renal insufficiency (creatinine >1.5 mg/dl), coagulation disorders, increased extra-systoles, blood pressure over 220/110 mmHg, respiratory insufficiency and heart frequency over 120/min. There was no age limit.

Within 45 minutes, a loading dose of 500 ml 10% HES 200/0.5 and 500 ml electrolyte solution was infused. Afterwards, a long-term infusion of 1000 ml of each solution was given over 24 hours. At the same time, dopamine and dobutamine were infused with a ratio of 1:1 (Kulka and Tryba 1993). The dopamine/dobutamine dose was raised stepwise every 5 minutes by 1 µg/kg bw/min up to the maximum dose of 8 to 10 µg/kg bw/min. After one hour, a maintenance dose of 4 to 6 µg/kg bw/min was infused over 5 hours. At the occurrence of angina pectoris, low ST in the EKG, increasing extra-systoles, increase of pulse over 140/min or blood pressure over 220/100 the dose was reduced.

CO was measured using the thoracic bioimpedance method (NCCOM3, BoMed, Irvine, USA). TCD measurements were carried out with a Multidop-X device (DWL, Überlingen, Germany). Flow velocity in the middle cerebral artery was measured at a depth of 50 mm. Measured parameters included systolic (Vs), mean (Vm) and diastolic (Vd) flow velocity as well as the pulsatility index as an expression of the cerebral vascular resistance. For the computation of the correlations, the values at the time of the change in dopamine/dobutamine dose were used. To determine blood pressure, an automatic blood pressure measuring device (Sirecust 401, Siemens, Erlangen, Germany) was used.

The labor-intensive, simultaneous and continuous measurement of CO, blood pressure and TCD was only possible in 10 patients with an infarction that was less than 12 hours old. The data was recorded and analyzed using special software (Stoll et al. 1992).

Mean value and standard deviation was computed. Significances were determined with the Wilcoxon and Mann and Whitney test. Correlations and 95% confidence intervals were computed with the Spearman correlation coefficient (Altman 1991).

Results

Effect of Hemodynamics on Clinical Course

From the clinical course, it was possible to divide the patients into two groups:
Group 1: patients with immediate clinical improvement under the therapy (n=13)
Group 2: patients with delayed or no clinical improvement (n=11) (Table 3).

Table 3. Clinical data of 24 patients with acute stroke treated with a sympathomimetically supported volume therapy divided in a group with improvement under the therapy (n=13) and a group with delayed or no clinical improvement (n=11)

	Group 1 (Improvement)	Group 2 (No improvement)
Age of patients	57	67
Initial score	26	56
Onset of therapy (h)	9.6	7.6
Risk factors		
Hypertension	5	5
Absolute arrhythmia	2	3
Diabetes	4	4
Smoking	5	3
Hyperlipidemia	6	6
Type of infarction		
Territorial	5	10
Lacunar	5	0
Hemodynamic	1	1
No CT demarcation	2	0

Patients in group 1 were younger, their neurological deficits less severe and their cardiovascular parameters better. Initial CO in group 1 was 7 l/min, in the other group 5 l/min. Initial heart frequency was lower in group 1 at 78/min than in the group without clinical improvement (105/min). Initial stroke volume in group 1 was 92 ml, in the second group 49 ml. Initial blood pressure in group 1 was 145/85 mmHg, in the second group 154/94 mmHg. The cardiovascular parameters confirm the clinical observation that patients without improvement had a limited cardiac competence.

Under the therapy, patients with clinical improvement showed a significant ($p < 0.01$) increase of CO and heart frequency by 30%, blood pressure rose by 10% (Fig. 8). Patients without clinical improvement showed an increase in hemodynamics that was only half as large (Fig. 9). Furthermore, this patient group reached earlier the therapy-limiting heart frequency over 120/min, so that they received a lower dopamine/dobutamine dose on average (Fig. 10). Due to the continuous monitoring and individual adjustment of dosages, no clinically relevant complications occurred.

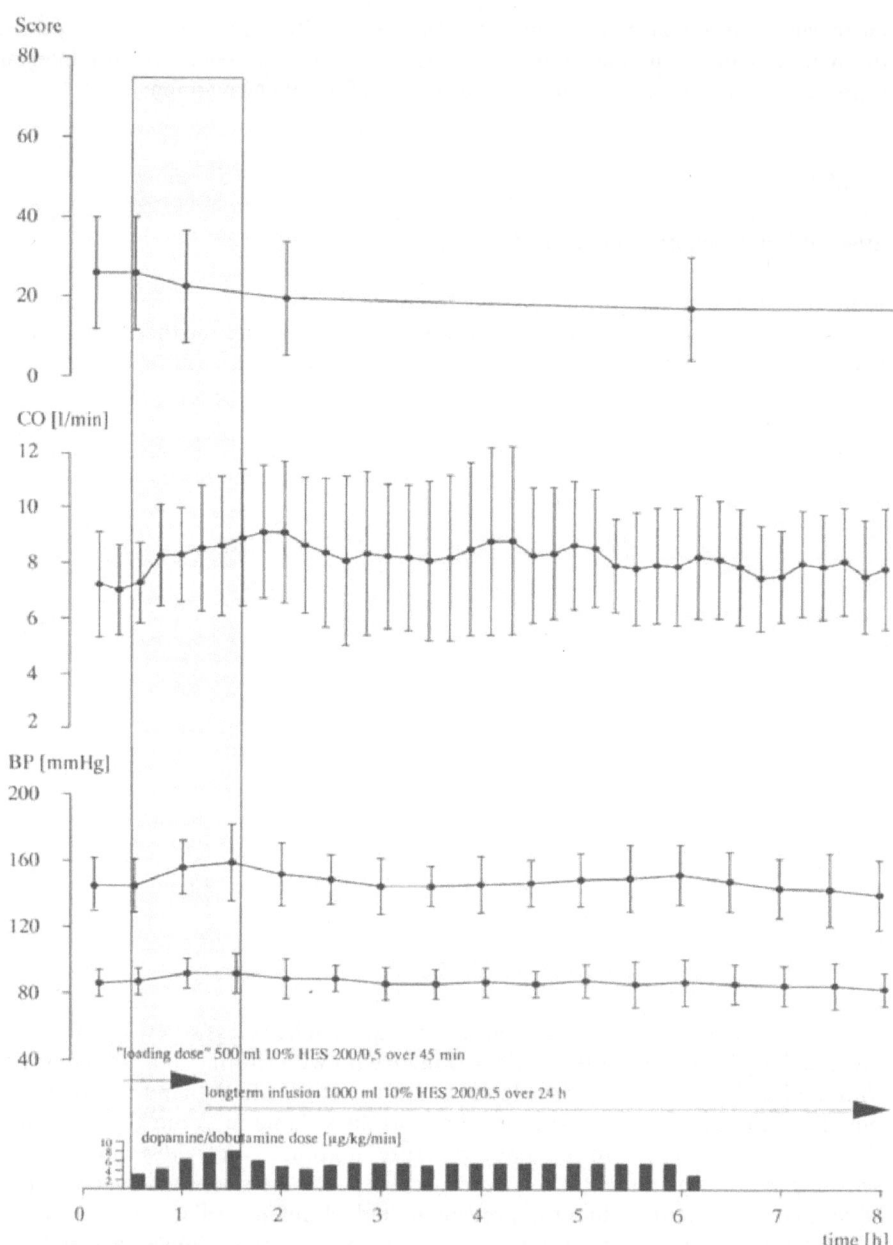

Fig. 8. Neurological score, CO, systolic and diastolic blood pressure (BP) of 13 patients with clinical improvement under a sympathomimetically supported volume therapy

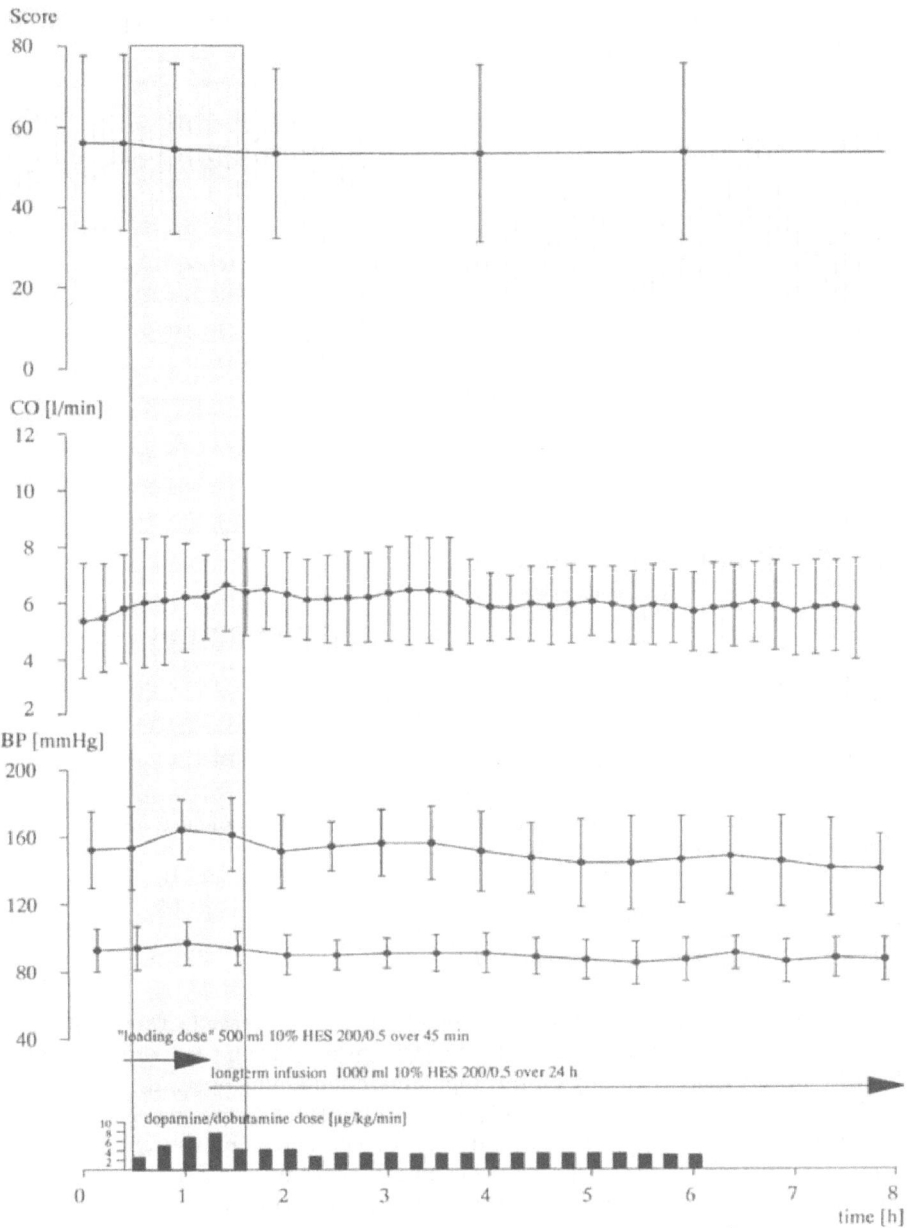

Fig. 9. Neurological score, CO, systolic and diastolic blood pressure (BP) of 11 patients without clinical improvement under a sympathomimetically supported volume therapy

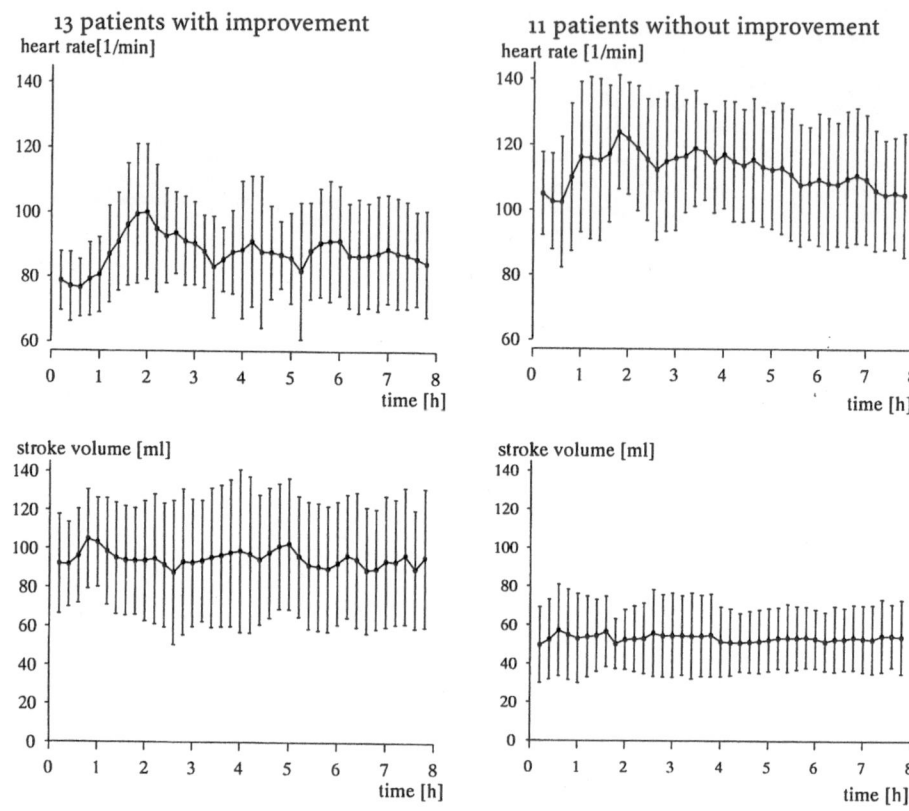

Fig. 10. Heart rate and stroke volume of 13 patients with and 11 patients without clinical improvement under sympathomimetically supported volume therapy

Effect of Hemodynamics on Cerebral Flow Velocity

The sympathomimetically supported volume therapy increased CO significantly in the 10 patients that were monitored with TCD (p<0.01) from 5.8 ± 1.3 l/min to 8.9 ± 2.2 l/min (Fig. 11), depending on the dopamine/dobutamine dose. At the same time, blood pressure increased from 139/84 to 156/93 mmHg. As expected, a close correlation existed between systolic, mean and diastolic blood pressure (r=0.92-0.96; p<0.01). Mean blood pressure was used for the computation of the correlations. The correlation between blood pressure and CO was only moderate (r=0.43; p<0.01). PI increased significantly in the un-affected hemisphere from 0.96 ± 0.09 to 1.41 ± 0.12 and in the affected hemisphere from 0.94 ± 0.06 to 1.37 ± 0.22. The PI values of the affected region were also consistently lower than the values of the contralateral side, however without reaching statistical significance.

Under therapy, Vs increased in the un-affected side from 95.8 ± 18.2 cm/s to 121.3 ± 23.8 cm/s (Fig. 12). The affected side showed an increase from 72.1 ± 26 cm/s to 80.2 ± 34.8 cm/s. This increase in Vs was significant in both groups (p<0.01). The

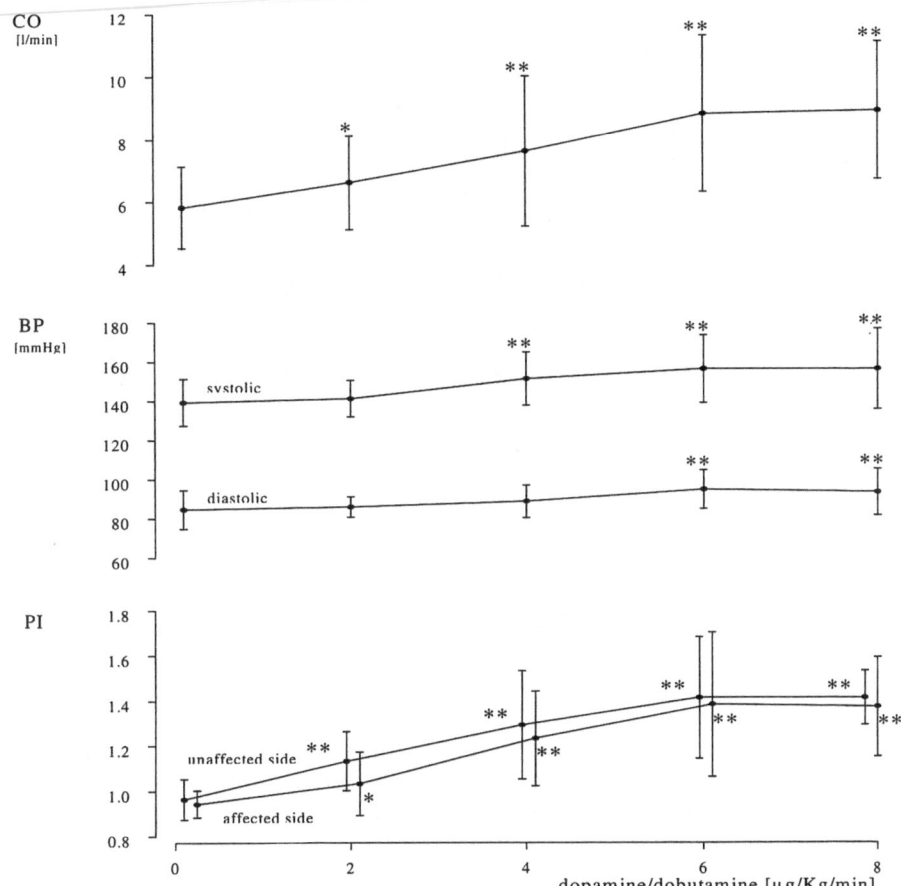

Fig. 11. CO, blood pressure (BP) and TCD pulsatility index (PI) in 10 patients with acute ischemic infarction in the region of the middle cerebral artery, depending on the dopamine/dobutamine dose (* p<0.05, ** p<0.01) (modified from Treib et al. 1996)

comparison between the hemispheres was also significant. Initial Vm in the affected side was at 44.8 ± 15.7 cm/s significantly (p<0.01) lower than in the other side (59.6 ± 12.1. cm/s). During the therapy, no significant changes in Vm occurred that correlated with the dopamine/dobutamine dose. Vd was in the affected hemisphere initially significantly (p<0.05) lower than in the un-affected side (30.1 ± 11.6 cm/s vs. 40.3 ± 9.5 cm/ s). Under the sympathomimetically supported volume therapy, both sides showed a small decline in Vd. At the time of the highest dopamine/dobutamine dose, Vd was 23.8 ± 9.4 cm/s and 35.7 ± 7.7 cm/s, respectively.

Computation of the correlations between the individual parameters showed the closest correlation exists between CO and PI in the affected (r=0.68) and in the un-affected (r=0.62) side (Fig. 13). The correlation between blood pressure and PI was lower, at 0.48 and 0.38, respectively.

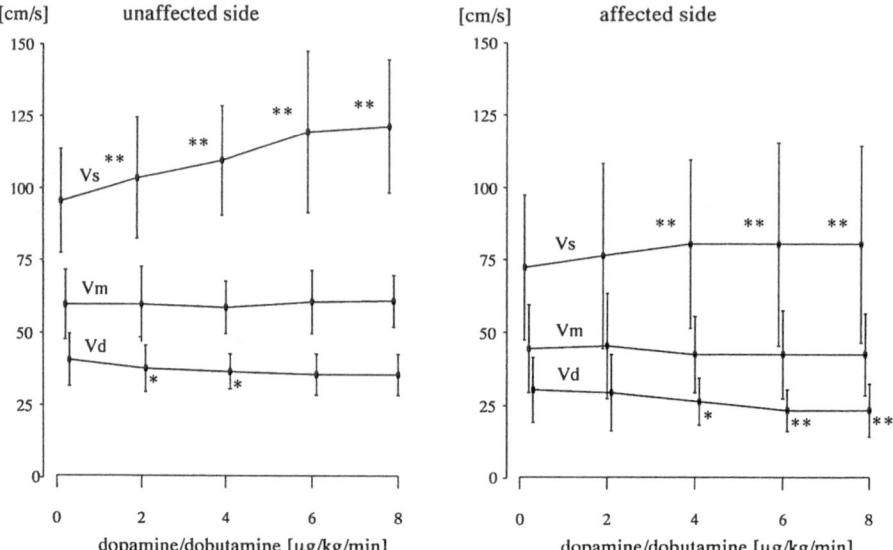

Fig. 12. Systolic (Vs), mean (Vm) and diastolic (Vd) TCD flow velocity in the affected and un-affected vascular region of 10 patients with an acute ischemic infarction in the region of the middle cerebral artery, in dependence of the dopamine/dobutamine dose (* $p<0.05$, ** $p<0.01$) (modified from Treib et al. 1996)

There was no correlation between Vm and CO in the un-affected side, nor a correlation between Vm and blood pressure (Fig. 14). The affected side showed a significant correlation between Vm and blood pressure, the correlation between Vm and CO showed a trend that was statistically not significant.

No patient suffered a clinical deterioration under the therapy. No respiratory or disorders of consciousness occurred. Repeatedly taken capillary blood gas analysis showed normal O_2 and CO_2 values.

Discussion

Currently, no scientifically validated data is available that supports the choice of a certain sympathomimetic agent for a hemodynamically oriented volume therapy. Although the pharmacological properties of catecholamines have been extensively studied in cardiologic patients, the corresponding studies are in general limited to cardiac patients with a low-output syndrome.

Contrary to cardiologic indications, sympathomimetically supported volume therapy attempts to increase cardiovascular parameters of patients with sufficient cardiovascular health above the normal range. A comparable therapeutic concept has been pursued by Shoemaker et al., who examined in a randomized study the effect of dopamine and dobutamine on the cardiovascular parameters of critically ill surgical patients (Shoemaker et al. 1989). In this study, dopamine lead to a larger increase in mean arterial blood pressure than dobutamine, whereas dobutamine raised

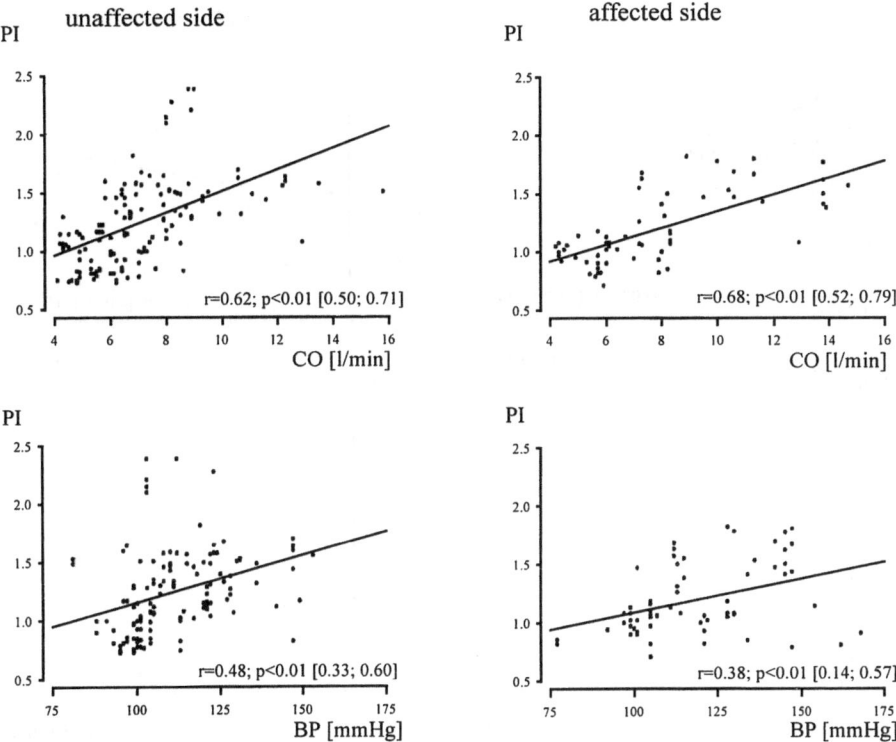

Fig. 13. Correlation between TCD pulsatility index (PI) and CO and mean blood pressure (BP) in the affected and unaffected vascular region of 10 patients with an acute infarction in the region of the middle cerebral artery, that were treated with sympathomimetically supported volume therapy (modified from Treib et al. 1996)

heart frequency and CO more. At the same time, dobutamine lowered wedge pressure and systemic vascular resistance more than dopamine. These effects can be explained through differing alpha- and beta-adrenergic effects of these drugs (Levy et al. 1993) (Table 4).

Table 4. Effects of dopamine, dobutamine an isoproterenol (modified from Levy et al. 1993)

Drug	Arrhythmia	i.v. dose (µg/kgbw/min)	Alpha-adrenergic	Beta-adrenergic
Dopamine	Moderate	1-4	Weak	Weak
		4-20	strong	moderate
Dobutamine	Weak	2-20	Weak	Strong
Isoproterenol	Strong	2-10	No	Strong

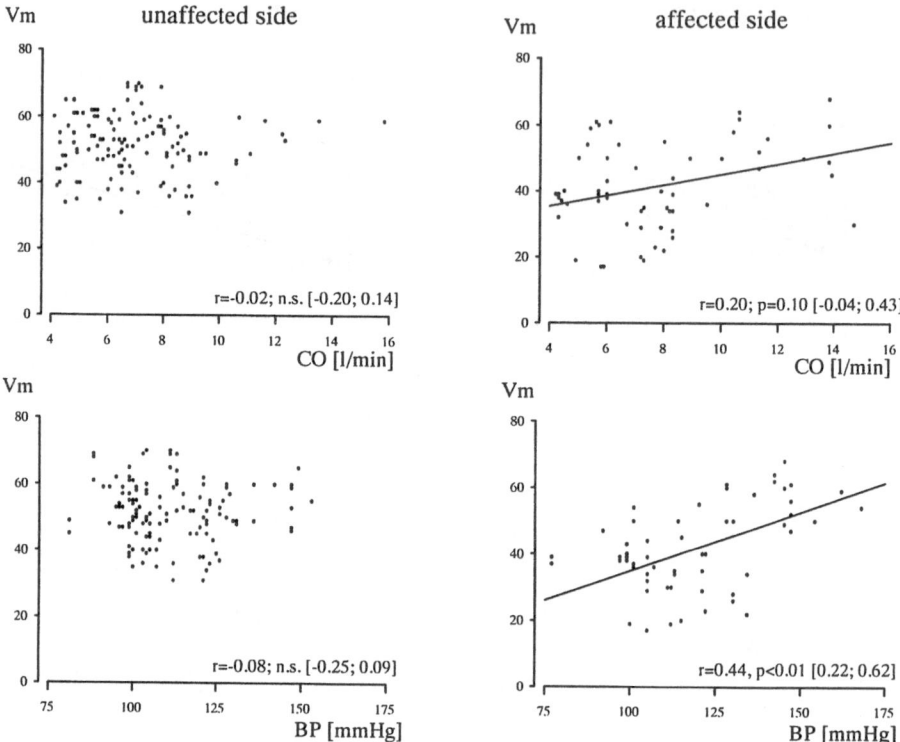

Fig. 14. Correlation between mean TCD flow velocity (Vm) and CO and mean blood pressure (BP) in in the affected and unaffected vascular region of 10 patients with an acute infarction in the region of the middle cerebral artery, that were treated with sympathomimetically supported volume therapy (modified from Treib et al. 1996)

One has to take into account that dopamine at lower doses increases renal perfusion and urine production, so that insufficient fluid intake can lead to hypovolemia. Because of the danger of arrhythmias, isoproterenol is hardly used.

Since Shoemaker et al. (1982, 1988, 1989, 1990) aimed for an increase of CO with blood pressure in the normal range, they preferred for their surgical patients dobutamine. Dobutamine causes fewer arrhythmias and has better effects on coronary perfusion and myocardial oxygen delivery than dopamine.

Contrary to surgical patients, stroke patients are not in need of an improvement of peripheral perfusion but need an improvement of the perfusion of ischemic brain regions. For this reason both, an increase of CO and an increase in blood pressure seem to be a reasonable way to increase cerebral perfusion pressure.

Because of the positive clinical results of Otsubo et al. (1990) in the treatment of vasospasm after subarachnoid hemorrhage, we combined the administration of dobutamine and dopamine to achieve an additional alpha-adrenergic effect.

The combination therapy dopamine/dobutamine chosen by us lead to a rapid clinical improvement in about half of the patients. 11 of 24 patients showed no clinical improvement. This group also showed no comparable increase of CO and blood pressure. The lacking therapeutic success can be attributed to a pre-existing limitation of cardiac competence. Indicators for this are the low initial CO and stroke volume, the higher initial heart frequency, higher blood pressure and higher age. Patients without clinical improvement also had more severe neurological deficits, in some cases complete infarctions in the region of the middle cerebral artery. In patients with a complete occlusion of the main stem of the medial cerebral artery, sufficient collateral supply is probably not possible, so that in these cases the existence of a penumbra is questionable. When a collateral supply is missing, the ischemic brain tissue becomes irreversibly damaged within minutes, and no therapeutic effect can be expected in these patients. This hypothesis is based on the experiences gathered during thrombolysis treatment of stroke (von Kummer et al. 1993).

Despite a comparable increase in hemodynamics, the share of our patients with clinical improvement (54%) was lower than in comparable vasospasm therapies, where in 70% to 78% of the cases a reduction of neurological benefits was observed (Otsubo et al. 1990, Levy et al. 1993). We attribute this to the fact that duration of therapy and observation was shorter in our study. Also, the therapeutic window in vasospasm is probably larger, because of the existing remaining perfusion.

The present study also yielded new results about the effects of hemodynamics on TCD flow velocity. TCD supplies information about direction of flow and flow velocity of the basal brain vessels. From the envelope curve of the frequency-time spectrum Vs, Vm and Vd can be computed. PI can be computed according to Gosling (1971) using the formula (Vs-Vd)/Vm = PI. PI depends on cerebral vascular resistance and is influenced by circulatory parameters, blood gases, elasticity of the blood vessels and intracranial pressure (ICP) (Giulioni et al. 1988, Chan et al. 1992). In healthy humans, PI ranges from 0.5 to 1.1 (Rath and Richter 1993). PI is clinically relevant particularly in patients with increased ICP (Treib et al. 1998). With increasing ICP, the flow profile becomes more pointed. During the diastole, flow velocity and therefore Vd, drops rapidly. Pulsatility and PI increase. When ICP reaches systemic diastolic arterial pressure, Vd becomes zero. When ICP continues to increase beyond this point, pendulum flow occurs and later systolic flow ceases (Hassler et al. 1988).

In several recent studies, a close correlation between ICP and PI was found (Felges und Mehdorn 1990, Cardoso and Kupchak 1992, Muttaqin et al. 1993). Inter-individual variability of PI is relatively large in patients with increased ICP (Treib et al. 1998). Intraindividually however, a close linear correlation between ICP and PI exists in the clinically relevant range (<60 mmHg) (Homburg et al. 1993, Rath und Richter 1993). Using TCD, it is therefore possible to gauge ICP, and when cardiovascular parameters and blood gases are constant, PI can be used intraindividually to monitor pressure-lowering therapy (Becker et al. 1996, Treib et al. 1998). Homburg and colleagues (1993) observed in healthy subjects a negative, exponential correlation between PI and partial pressure of CO_2. They did not describe the effects of CO and blood pressure on PI.

In our study, the hemodynamic increase resulted in both hemispheres in a comparable increase of PI. Three possible mechanisms could explain this increase of almost 50%.

1. Dopamine and dobutamine cause a vasoconstriction of the cerebral vessels
2. Raising CO and blood pressure causes an increase of ICP
3. The autoregulation of the cerebral vessels counteracts the increase in CO and blood pressure

1. The fact that the therapy did not affect Vm does not support the hypothesis of a pharmacogenic vasoconstriction in the area of the middle cerebral artery. It is known that Vm increases during vasospasm in subarachnoid hemorrhage (Sekhar et al. 1988, Lindegaard et al. 1989). However, vasoconstriction in the peripheral small vessels could lead to an increase of PI.

2. An increased PI has been observed in patients suffering from increased ICP (Felges and Mehdorn 1990, Homburg et al. 1993, Muttaqin et al. 1993). The effects of a sympathomimetically supported hypervolemic hemodilution on ICP have not been studied so far. Nau and colleagues (1992) measured after infusion of dopamine a drop in patients with mildly elevated ICP and an increase of ICP in patients with strongly elevated ICP. Wood and colleagues (1983) observed in animal experiments after excessive hypervolemic hemodilution a slight increase in ICP of about 5 mmHg, whereas Lyden et al. (1988) did not observe a hemodilution-induced increase in ischemic brain edema. In the studies discussed, the significant increase of Vs speaks against an increase of ICP, because when ICP increases, one would expect a drop of Vd, with Vs remaining almost constant (Cardoso and Kupchak 1992, Homburg et al. 1993). One limitation however has to be considered: this holds only true if cardiovascular parameters remain constant, which was not the case in the present study. The fact that PI in the ischemic hemisphere was always lower than on the other side is another argument against therapy-induced increase in ICP. If as a result of the growing ischemic brain edema local ICP grows, PI increase should be higher on the affected side. Overall, it cannot be excluded that sympathomimetically supported volume therapy can cause a small increase in ICP. Nevertheless, the 50% increase of PI in our study cannot be explained through an increase in ICP, because there were no clinical signs for a manifest, therapy-induced increase ICP.

3. In our opinion, the flow velocity changes observed by TCD can be best explained through a counteraction of the cerebral autoregulation, induced by elevated CO and blood pressure. In earlier studies, we were able to show that volume alone does not lead to a constant increase of CO and blood pressure. This explains why Volc and colleagues did not measure a change in PI with hemodilution therapy alone (Volc et al. 1995). Through the additional infusion of dopamine and dobutamine, we achieved in our current study a pronounced improvement of hemodynamics. The therapy-induced increase in blood pressure was relatively small at 12% and does not explain the observed effects on Vs and PI satisfactorily. The percentage increase in CO corresponds roughly to the increase in PI. The association between these two parameters has not been studied sufficiently.

The therapy-induced increase in PI should, according to animal studies by Tranmer et al. (1986), have a favorable influence on blood flow of the ischemic brain regions. After occluding the middle cerebral artery, the authors noted that local cerebral blood flow in the ischemic regions grew by 55%, when extracorporal perfusion was changes from non-pulsatile to pulsatile flow. Concurrently, a significant improvement of the electro-encephalographic mapping-power analysis occurred. By contrast, the authors observed only a 19% increase in local blood flow in the non-ischemic regions.

The correlations computed by us show a weaker correlation between blood pressure and PI than between CO and PI, both in the affected and un-affected hemisphere

(Fig. 13). This result suggests that CO has a greater impact on cerebro-vascular resistance than blood pressure.

Regarding Vm, there was no correlation between Vm and CO or Vm and blood pressure in the un-affected hemisphere. Because according to the studies by Saha et al. 1993 such correlation should not exist when autoregulation is intact, the fact that the correlation values are almost zero show the validity of the method. However, in ischemia-impaired autoregulation, a correlation existed, which was closer between Vm and blood pressure than between Vm and CO (Fig. 14).

The present study suggests that cerebral perfusion and autoregulation of the patient with acute stroke do not only depend on perfusion pressure, but also on CO. The moderate correlation of 0.45 indicates that CO and blood pressure do not depend directly on each other. This is important in the therapy of acute stroke as well as for vasospasm therapy of patients with subarachnoid hemorrhage. In the hyperdynamic therapy of these disorders, the physician should not only pay attention to increasing blood pressure, but also to CO. The thoracic bioimpedance method is hereby suitable for non-invasive monitoring.

Pathophysiological research and the results of animal studies suggest that the ischemic penumbra, which is limited in its auto-regulative counteractions, profits from an increase in CO and blood pressure. Because autoregulation is impaired, any hemodynamic improvement is directly passed on to the penumbra (Davis et al. 1980, Keller et al. 1982, Werner et al. 1991, Tranmer et al. 1992, Ohtaki and Tranmer 1993). Moreover, the therapy-induced auto-regulative increase in vascular resistance of the surrounding, un-affected brain tissue will increase relative supply for the penumbra, because the increase in CO and blood pressure is focused on the penumbra. This hypothesis is supported by the fact that the hemodynamic increase was accompanied by simultaneous clinical improvement in more than half of the patients.

Because of the highly variable course of cerebral perfusion disorders, the clinical efficacy of sympathomimetically-supported volume therapy can only be proven in a large, randomized study. Should the hemodynamic therapy concept prove to be effective, it could improve the outcome of brain strokes in combination with other therapies such as fibrinolysis or calcium antagonists, rheological drugs, nootropics or neuroprotectiva substances (Kempski 1994, Wityk et al. 1994).

References

Adams RJ, Meador KJ, Sethi KD, Grotta JC, Thomson DS: Graded neurologic scale for use in acute hemispheric stroke treatment protocols. Stroke 18, 665-669, 1987

Adams HP, Brott TG, Crowell RM, Furlan AJ, Gomez CR, Grotta J, Helgason CM, Marler JR, Woolson RF, Zivin JA, Feinberg W, Mayberg M: Guidelines for the management of patients with acute ischemic stroke. Stroke 25, 1901-1914, 1994

Aichner FT, Fazekas F, Brainin M, Pölz W, Mamoli B, Zeiler K: Hypervolemic hemodilution in acute stroke. The multicenter Austrian hemodilution stroke trial (MAHST). Stroke 29, 743-749, 1998

Altman DG: Practical statistics for medical research. Chapman and Hall, London, 1991

Appel PL, Kram HB, MacKabee J, Fleming AW, Shoemaker WC: Comparison of measurements of cardiac output by bioimpedance and thermodilution in severely ill surgical patients. Crit Care Med 14, 933-935, 1986

Aspey BS, Ehteshami S, Hurst CM, McCoy AL, Harrison MJG: The effect of increased blood pressure on hemisperic lactate and water content during acute cerebral ischaemia in the rat and gerbil. J Neurol Neurosurg Psychiat 50, 1493-1498, 1987

Back T, von Kummer R: Blutverdünnung bei zerebraler Ischämie. Abschied von einem verbreiteten Behandlungskonzept. Dtsch med Wschr 114, 350-356, 1989

Becker S, Hassler M, Treib J, Haaß A, Schimrigk K: Transkranielle Dopplersonographie zur Überwachung der Hirnödemtherapie. In: Treib J, Stoll M, Lindemuth R (Hrsg) Abstracts der 13. Arbeitstagung der Arbeitsgemeinschaft für Neurologische Intensivmedizin. Conrad und Bothner, Zweibrücken, 146, 1996

Bernstein DP: A new stroke volume equation for thoracic electrical bioimpedance: Theory and rationale. Crit Care Med 14, 904-909, 1986

Bernstein DP: Continuous noninvasive real-time monitoring of stroke volume and cardiac output by thoracic electrical bioimpedance. Crit Care Med 14, 898-901, 1986

Bladin CF, Chambers BR: Frequency and pathogenesis of hemodynamic stroke. Stroke 25, 2179-2182, 1994

Boldt J, Kling D, Thiel A, Hempelmann G: Nicht-invasive versus invasive Kreislaufüberwachung. Bestimmung des Herzzeitvolumens und des pulmonalen Hydrationszustandes mit Hilfe eines neuen Bioimpedanz-Monitors. Anaesthesist 37, 218-223, 1988

Boyd O, Grounds M, Bennet D: A randomized clinical trial of the effect of deliberate perioperative increase of oxygen delivery on mortality in high-risk surgical patients. JAMA 270, 2699-2707, 1993

Bonita R: Epidemiology of stroke. Lancet 339, 342-344, 1992

Bonelli J, Jancuska M: Exsikkose im Alter. Wien Med Wschr 22, 487-490, 1984

Bouma GJ, Muizelaar JP: Relationship between cardiac output and cerebral blood flow in patients with intact and with impaired autoregualtion. J Neurosurg 73, 368-374, 1990

Britton M, Carlsson A, De Faire U: Blood pressure course in patients with acute stroke and matched controls. Stroke 17, 861-864, 1986

Britton M, Carlsson A: Very high blood pressure in acute stroke. J Intern Med 228, 611-615, 1990

Broderick J, Brott T, Barsan W, Haley EC, Levy D, Marler J, Sheppard G, Blum C: Blood pressure during the first minutes of focal cerebral ischemia. Ann Emerg Med 22, 1438-1443, 1993

Brunner FP: Pathophysiologie der Dehydratation. Schweiz Rundschau Med 82, 784-787, 1993

Cardoso ER, Kupchak JA: Evaluation of intracranial pressure gradients by means of transcranial doppler sonography. Acta Neurochir 55, Suppl., 1-5, 1992

Carlberg B, Asplund K, Hägg E: Factors influencing admission blood pressure levels in patients with acute stroke. Stroke 22, 527-530, 1991

Castor G, Altmayer P, Molter G, Müller D, Simon J: Herzzeitvolumenmessung mittels nichtinvasiver elektrischer Bioimpedanz im Vergleich zur Thermodilutionsmethode. Anästh Intensivmed 29, 339-344, 1988

Castor G, Altmayer P, Molter G, Helms J, Bach R, Simon J: Eine neue nichtinvasive Methode zur kontinuierlichen Bestimmung der linksventrikulären Ejektionsfraktion. Intensivmed 26, 488-490, 1989

Castor G, Molter G, Helms J, Niedermark I, Altmayer P: Determination of cardiac output during positive endexpiratory pressure – Noninvasive electrical bioimpedance compared with standard thermodilution. Crit Care Med 18, 544-546, 1990

Castor G, Klocke RK, Stoll M, Helms J, Niedermark I: Simultaneous measurement of cardiac output by thermodilution, thoracic electrical bioimpedance and doppler ultrasound. Br J Anaesth 72, 133-138, 1994

Chan K-W, Miller JD, Dearden NM, Andrews PJD, Midglen SM: The effect of changes in cerebral perfusion pressure upon middle cerebral artery blood flow velocity and jugular bulb venous oxygen saturation after severe brain injury. J Neurosurg. 77, 55-61, 1992

Clancy TV, Norman K, Reynolds R, Covington D, Maxwell JG: Cardiac output measurement in critical care patients: Thoracic electrical bioimpedance versus thermodilution. J Trauma 31, 1116-1121, 1991

van Daele ME, Trouwborst A, van Woerkens LC, Tenbrinck R, Fraser AG, Roelandt JR: Transesophageal echocardiographic monitoring of preoperative acute hypervolemic hemodilution. Anaesthesiology 81, 602-609, 1994

Davis DH, Sundt TM: Relationship of cerebral blood flow to cardiac output, mean arterial pressure, blood volume, and alpha and beta blockade in cats. J Neurosurg 52, 745-754, 1980

Dandapani BK, Suzuki S, Kelly RE, Reyes-Iglesias Y, Duncan RC: Relation between blood pressure and outcome in intracerebral hemorrhage. Stroke 26, 21-24, 1995 de Deyn PP: The piracetam in acute stroke study. Eur J Neurol 2, 7, 1995

European Atrial Fibrillation Trial Study Group. Secondary prevention in non-rheumatic atrial fibrillation after transient ischaemic attack or minor stroke. Lancet 342, 1255-1262, 1993

European Cooperative Acute Stroke Study (ECASS). Intravenous thrombolysis with recombinant tissue plasminogen activator for acute hemispheric stroke. JAMA 274, 1017-1025, 1995

European Carotid Surgery Trialists Collaborative Group: MRC European Carotid Surgery Trial: interim results for symptomatic patients with severe (70-99%) or with mild (0-29%) carotid stenosis. Lancet 337, 1235-1243, 1991

Felges A, Mehdorn HM: Zum Einsatz der transkraniellen Dopplersonographie auf einer neurochirurgischen Intensivstation. Wien Med Wschr 24, 567-570, 1990

Fenske A, Kohl J, Regli F, Reulen HJ: The effect of arterial hypertenion on focal ischemic edema. J Neurol 219, 241-251, 1978

Fujii K, Sadoshima S, Okada Y, Yao H, Kuwabara Y, Ichiya Y, Fujishima M: Cerebral blood flow and metabolism in normotensive and hypertensive patients with transient neurologic deficits. Stroke 21, 283-290, 1990

Gabler-Sandberger E: Die Helsingborg-Deklaration. Richtlinien zur Therapie des Apoplex. Dtsch Ärztebl 93, 132-133, 1996

Gent M, Blakely JA, Easton JD, Ellis DJ, Hachinski VC, Harbison JW, Panak E, Roberts RS, Sicurella J, Turpie AGG: The Canadian American Ticlopidine Study (Cats) in thromboembolic stroke. Lancet I, 1215-1220, 1989

Giulioni M, Ursino M, Alvisi C: Correlations among intracranial pulsatility, intracranial hemodynamics, and transcranial doppler wave form: Literature review and hypothesis for future studies. Neurosurgery 22, 807-812, 1988

Goldstein DS, Cannon RO, Zimlichman R, Keiser HR: Clinical evaluation of impedance cardiography. Clinical Physiology 6, 235-251, 1986

Goldstein RA, Passamani ER, Roberts R: A comparison of digoxin and dobutamine in patients with acute infarction and cardiac failure. N Engl J Med 303, 846-850, 1980

Gosling RG, Dunbar G, King DH, Newman DL, Side CD, Woodcock JP, Fitzgerald DE, Keates JS, MacMillan D: The quantitative analysis of occlusive peripheral arterial disease by a non-intrusive ultrasonic technique. Angiology 22, 52-55, 1971

Goslinga H, Eijzenbach V, Heuvelmans JHA, van der Laan de Vries E, Melis VMJ, Schmid-Schönbein H, Bezemer PD: Custom-tailored hemodilution with albumin and crystalloids in acute ischemic stroke. Stroke 23, 181-188, 1992

Gottstein U: Physiologie und Pathophysiologie des Hirnkreislaufs. Med Welt 15, 715-726, 1965

Gottstein U, Held K: Effekt der Hämodilution nach intravenöser Infusion von niedermolekularen Dextranen auf die Hirnzirkulation des Menschen. Dtsch Med Wschr 11, 522-526, 1969

Gottstein U: Hemodilution therapy in acute ischemic stroke. In: Kriegelstein J (ed) Pharmacology of cerebral ischemia. Elsevier Science Publisher, 221-229, 1986

Grauer MT, Woessner R, Haaß A, Treib J: Volume therapy in patients with acute stroke. Transfusion Alternatives in Transfusion Medicine (TATM), in press

Grossmann W: Akute zerebrale Ischämie. Praktische Diagnostik und erste therapeutische Maßnahmen. Münch Med Wschr 125, 323-327, 1983

Grotta JC, Pettigrew LC, Allen S, Tonnesen A, Yatsu FM, Gray J, Spydell J: Baseline hemodynamic state and response to hemodilution in patients with acute cerebral ischemia. Stroke 16, 790-795, 1985

Grotta JC: Current status of hemodilution in acute cerebral ischemia. Stroke 18, 689-690, 1987

Haaß A, Kroemer H, Jäger H, Oest A, Heinrich B: Hemodilution therapie in cerebral ischemia, different dose- and timedependent hemorheological effects of plasma expanders. In: Kriegelstein J (ed): Pharmacology of cerebral ischemia. Elsevier, Amsterdam, 1986

Haaß A, Kroemer H, Jäger H, Müller K, Decker I, Wagner EM, Schimrigk K: Dextran 40 oder HES 200/0,5 ? Hämorheologie der Langzeitbehandlung beim ischämischen zerebralen Insult. Dtsch Med Wschr 111, 1681-1686, 1986

Haaß A, Kroemer H, Jäger H, Oest A, Schimrigk K: Similar and opposite hemorheological effects of dextran 40 and hydroxyethyl starch in hemodilution therapie for stroke. In: Hartmann A and Kuschinsky W (eds.): Cerebral ischemia and hemorheology. Springer, Berlin-Heidelberg, 1987

Haaß A: Hämodilution mit mittelmolekularer Stärke zur Therapie des ischämischen Insultes, der Subarachnoidalblutung und intrazerebralen Blutung, hämorheologische und gerinnungsphysiologische Probleme. In: Lawin P (Hrsg): Hydroxyäthylstärke, eine aktuelle Übersicht. Thieme, Stuttgart New York, 1989

Haaß A: Therapie des akuten ischämischen Insultes. Nervenheilkunde 8, 35-45, 1989

Haaß A: Hämorheologische Therapie, Stand und Perspektiven. Nervenarzt 60, 528-539, 1989

Haaß A: Hämodilutionstherapie beim ischämischen Hirninfarkt: Sinnvoll. Akt Neurol 16, 213-219, 1989

Haaß A, Stoll M, Treib J: Hämodilution bei cerebralen Durchblutungsstörungen. Indikation, Durchführung, medikamentöse Zusatzbehandlung und Alternativen. In: Koscielny J, Kiesewetter H, Jung F, Haaß A (Hrsg): Hämodilution, neue Aspekte in der Behandlung von Durchblutungsstörungen. Springer, Berlin-Heidelberg, 1991

Haaß A, Stoll M, Treib J, Krack P, Decker I, Hamann G, Kässer U: Hämorheologische und hämodynamische Befunde und ihre klinische Bedeutung für die Hämodilution. In: Landgraf H, Ehrly AM (Hrsg): Hämodilution bei akuter zerebraler Ischämie. Blackwell Wissenschaft, Berlin, 1992

Haaß A, Treib J, Stoll M: Hemorheological parameters of hydroxyethyl starch 200/0,62 as a basis for hemodilution. Clin Hemorheol 12, Supp. 1, 17-26, 1992

Haaß A: Hemorheological risc factors for ischemic stroke. In: Dorndorf W, Marx P (eds) Stroke prevention. Karger, Basel 53-66, 1994

Hamann G: Hormonelle, autonome Veränderungen bei lebensbedrohlichen intrakraniellen Erkrankungen. Klinische und biochemische Ergebnisse zur zerebralen Streßreaktion. Habilitationsschrift, Homburg, 1993

Hankey GJ, Gubbay SS: Focal cerebral ischaemia and infarction due to antihypertensive therapy. Med J Aust 20, 412-414, 1987

Harper AM: Autoregulation of cerebral blood flow: Influence of the arterial blood pressure on the blood flow through the cortex. J Neurol Neurosurg Psychiat 29, 398-403, 1966

Harrison MJG, Pollock S, Kendall BE, Marshall J: Effect of haematokrit on carotid stenosis and cerebral infarction. Lancet II, 114-115, 1981

Harrison MJG: Protection against ischemia: the basis of acute stroke therapy. Curr Opin Neurol Neurosurg 5, 33-38, 1992

Hassler W, Steinmetz H, Gawlowski J: Transcranial doppler ultrasonography in raised intracranial pressure and in intracranial circulatory arrest. J Neurosurg 68, 745-751, 1988

Heber H, Kolde HJ, Heimburger N, Svendsen G: New chromogenic substrate for C1-inhibitor functional activity assay. Thromb Haemost 50, 227, 1983

Heiß W-D: Prävemtion, Diagnostik und Therapie des ischänischen Insults. Dt Ärztebl 93, 653-656, 1996

Hemodilution in stroke study group: Hypervolemic hemodilution treatment of acute stroke, results of a randomized multicenter trial using pentastarch. Stroke 20, 317-323, 1989

Hino A, Ueda S, Mizukawa N, Imahori Y, Tenjin H: Effect of hemodilution on cerebral hemodynamics and oxygen metabolism. Stroke 23, 423-426, 1992

Homburg AM, Jakobsen M, Enevoldsen E: Transcranial doppler recordings in raised intracranial pressure. Acta Neurol Scand 87, 488-493, 1993

Indredavic B, Bakke F, Solberg R, Rokseth R, Haaheim LL, Holme I: Benefit of a stroke unit: a randomized controlled trial. Stroke 22, 1026-1031, 1991

Introna RPS, Pruett JK, Crumrine RC: Use of transthoracic bioimpedance to determine cardiac output in pediatric patients. Crit Care Med 16, 1101-1105, 1988

Irie K, Yamaguchi T, Minematsu K, Omae T: The j-curve phenomenon in stroke recurrence. Stroke 24, 1844-1849, 1993

The Italian Acute Stroke Study Group: The Italian haemodilution trial in acute stroke. Stroke 18, 670-676, 1987

The Italian Acute Stroke Study Group: Haemodilution in acute stroke, results of the italian haemodilution trial. Lancet I, 318-321, 1988

Janzon L, Bergqvist D, Boberg J, Boberg M, Eriksson I, Lindgärde, Persson G: Prevention of myocardial infarction and stroke in patients with intermittent claudicatio; effects of Ticlopidine. Results from STIMS, the swedish Ticlopedine multicenter study. J Intern Med 227, 301-308, 1991

Jarisch A: Kreislauffragen. Dtsch Med Wschr 54, 1211-1213, 1928

Jörgensen HS, Nakayama H, Raaschou HO, Olsen TS: Effect of blood pressure and diabetes on stroke in progression. Lancet 344, 156-159, 1994

Kaste M, Fogelholm R, Erila T, Palomaki H, Murros K, Rissanen A, Sarna S: A randomized, double-blind, placebo-controlled trial of nimodipine in acute ischemic hemisheric stroke. Stroke 25, 1348-1353, 1994

Keller TS, McGillicuddy JE, LaBond VA, Kindt GW: Volume expansion in focal cerebral ischemia: the effect of cardiac output on local cerebral blood flow. Clin Neurosurg 29, 40-50, 1982

Kempski OS: Neuroprotektion, Modelle und Grundprinzipien. Anaesthesist 43, S23-S33, 1994

Kiesewetter H, Jung F, Blume J, Gerhards M: Hämodilution bei Patienten mit peripherer arterieller Verschlußkrankheit im Stadium IIb: Prospektiver randomisierter Doppelblind-Vergleich von mittelmolekularer Hydroxyäthylstärke und kleinmolekularer Dextranlösung. Klin Wschr 65, 324-330, 1987

Kiyohara Y, Fujishima M, Ishitsuka T, Tamaki K, Sadoshima S, Omae T: Effects of hematocrit on brain metabolism in experimental induced cerebral ischemia in spontaneously hypertensive rats (SHR). Stroke 16, 835-840, 1985

Kiyohara Y, Ueda K, Hasuo Y, Fujii I, Yanai T, Wada J, Kawano H, Shikata T, Omae T, Fujishima M: Hematocrit as a risc factor of cerebral infarction: Long term prospective population survey in a japanese rural community. Stroke 17, 687-692, 1986

Koller M, Haenny P, Hess K, Weniger D, Zangger P: Adjusted hypervolamic hemodilution in acute ischemic stroke. Stroke 21, 1429-1434, 1990

Koscielny J, Förster H, Kolepke W, Jung F: Vergleich von iso- und hypervolämischer Hämodilution mit HES. In: Koscielny J, Kiesewetter H, Jung F, Haaß A (Hrsg): Hämodilution, neue Aspekte in der Behandlung von Durchblutungsstörungen. Springer, Berlin Heidelberg New Nork, 146-228, 1991

Kulka PJ, Tryba M: Inotropic support of the critically ill patient. Drugs 45, 654-667, 1993

von Kummer R, Forsting M, Wildemann B, Sartor K: Thrombolyse bei akuter zerebraler Ischämie. Akt Radiol 3, 351-355, 1993

von Kummer R, Bozzao L, Manelfe C: Early CT Diagnosis of hemispheric brain infarction. Springer, Berlin Heidelberg New York, 1995

Kusunoki M, Kimura K, Nakamura M, Isaka Y, Yoneda S, Abe H: Effects of hematocrit variations on cerebral blood flow and oxygen transport in ischemic cerebrovascular disease. J Cereb Blood Flow Metab 1, 413-417, 1981

Langhorne P, Williams BO, Gilchrist W, Howie K: Do stroke units save lives ? Lancet 342, 395-398, 1993

Langhorne P, Dennis MS, Williams BO: Stroke units: their role in acute stroke management. Vasc Med Rev 6, 33-44, 1995

Lavin P: Management of hypertension in patients with acute stroke. Arch Intern Med 146, 66-68, 1986

Levy ML, Rabb CH, Zelman V, Giannotta SL: Cardiac performance enhancement from dobutamine in patients refractory to hypervolemic therapy for cerebral vasospasm. J Neurosurg 79, 494-499, 1993

Leys D, Mounier-Vehier F, Mounier-Vehier C, Carre A: Relationship between blood pressure and outcome in intracerebral hemorrhage. Stroke 26, 1126-1127, 1995

Lin S-Z, Chiou T-L, Chiang Y-H, Song W-S: Hemodilution accelerates the passage of plasma (not red cells) through cerebral microvessels in rats. Stroke 26, 2166-2171, 1995

Lowe GDO, Jaap AJ, Forbes CD: Relation of atrial fibrillation and high haematokrit to mortality in acute stroke. Lancet I, 784-786, 1983

Lindegaard K-F, Nornes H, Bakke SJ, Sorteberg W, Nakstad P: Cerebral vasospasm diagnosis by means of angiography and blood velocity measurements. Acta Neurochir (Wien) 100, 12-24, 1989

Lisk DR, Grotta JC, Lamki LM, Tran HD, Taylor JW, Molony DA, Barron BJ: Should hypertension be treated after acute stroke ? A randomized controlled trial using single photon emission computed tomography. Arch Neurol 50, 855-862, 1993

Lyden PD, Alving LI, Zivin JA, Rothrock JF: Hemodilution with low-molecular-weight hydroxyethyl starch after experimental focal cerebral ischemia in rats. Stroke 19, 223-227, 1988

Marmot MG, Poulter NR: Primary prevention of stroke. Lancet 339, 344-347, 1992

Marx P, Haaß A, Hartmann A: Hämodilutionsbehandlung des ischämischen Insultes. MMW 137, 147-150, 1995

Mast H, Marx P: Neurological deterioration under isovolemic hemodilution with hydroxyethyl starch in acute cerebral ischemia. Stroke 22, 680-683, 1991

Mast H, Marx P: Neurologische Verschlechterung unter Hämodilution bei zerebraler Ischämie. In: Landgraf H, Ehrly AM (ed.): Hämodilution bei akuter zerebraler Ischämie. Blackwell Wissenschaft, Berlin, 78-85, 1992

Mattar JA, Baruzzi ACA, Diament D, Szynkier RT, de Felippe J, da Luz PL, Auler JO, Lage S, Pileggi F, Jatene A: A clinical comparison between cardiac output measured by thermodilution versus noninvasive thoracic electrical bioimpedance. Acute Care 12, 58-60, 1986

Menger MD: Microcirculation disturbances secundary to ischemia-reperfusion. Transplantation Proceedings 27, 2863-2865, 1995

Millar-Craig MW, Bishop CN, Raftery EB: Circadian variation of blood-pressure. Lancet 795-797, 1978

Mori K, Arai H, Nakajima K, Tajima A, Maeda M: Hemorheological and hemodynamic analysis of hypervolemic hemodilution therapy for cerebral vasospasm after aneurysmal subarachnoid hemorrhage. Stroke 26, 1620-1626, 1995

Muttaqin Z, Uozumi T, Kuwabara S, Arita K, Kurisu K, Ohba S, Kohno H, Ogasawara H, Ohtani M, Mikami T: Hyperaemia prior to acute cerebral swelling in severe head injuries: the role of transcranial doppler monitoring. Acta Neurochir (Wien) 123, 76-81, 1993

Nau R, Sander D, Klingelhöfer J: Relationships between dopamine infusion and intracranial hemodynamics in patients with raised intracranial pressure. Clin Neurol Neurosurg 94, 143-148, 1992

North American Symptomatic Carotid Endarterectomy Trial (NASCET): Clinical Alert: Benefit of carotid endarterectomy for patients with high-grade stenosis of the internal carotid artery. Stroke 22, 816-817, 1991

Ohtaki M, Tranmer BI: Hyperdynamic therapy for focal cerebral ischemia in rats: use of colloidal volume expansion and dobutamine. Surg Neurol 40, 131-137, 1993

Otsubo H, Takemae T, Inoue T, Kobayahi S, Sugita K: Normovolaemic induced hypertension therapy for cerebral vasospasm after subarachnoid haemorrhage. Acta Neurochir Wien 103, 18-26, 1990

Olsen TS, Larsen B, Herning M, Skriver EB, Lassen NA: Blood flow and vascular reactivity in collaterally perfused brain tissue. Evidence of an ischemic penumbra in patients with acute stroke. Stroke 14, 332-341, 1983

Perez-Trepichio AD, Furlan AJ, Little JR, Jones SC: Hydroxyethyl starch 200/0,5 reduces infarct volume after embolic stroke in rats. Stroke 23, 1782-1790, 1992

Phillips PA, Johnston CI, Gray L: Disturbed fluid and electrolyte homoeostasis following dehydration in elderly people. Age Ageing 22, S26-33, 1993

Phillips PA, Rolls BJ, Ledingham JGG, Forsling ML, Morton JJ, Crowe MJ, Wollner L: Reduced thirst after water deprivation in healthy elderly men. N Engl J Med 311, 753-759, 1984

Powers WJ, Raichle ME: Positron emission tomography and its application to the study of the study of cerebrovascular disease in man. Stroke 16, 361-376, 1985

Pries AR, Fritzsche A, Ley K, Gaehtgens P: Redistribution of red blood cell flow in microcirculatory networks by hemodilution. Circ Res 70, 1113-1121, 1992

Pries AR, Neuhaus D, Gaehtgens P: Blood viscosity in tube flow: dependence on diameter and hematocrit. Am J Physiol 263, 1771-1778, 1992

Pries AR, Secomb TW, Gaehtgens P, Gross JF: Blood flow in microvascular networks. Experiments and simulation. Circ Res 67, 826-834, 1990

Pries AR, Secomb TW, Gaehtgens P: Structure and hemodynamics of microvascular networks: heterogenity and correlations. Am J Physiol 269, 1713-1722, 1995

Pries AR, Secomb TW, Gaehtgens P: Design principles of vascular beds. Circ Res 77, 1017-1023, 1995

Pries AR, Secomb TW, Geßner T, Sperandio MB, Gross JF, Gaehtgens P: Resistance to blood flow in microvessels in vivo. Circ Res 75, 904-915, 1994

Rath SA, Richter H-P: Die transkranielle Doppler-Sonographie als aussagefähiges Diagnostikum beim Schädel-Hirn-Trauma. Unfallchirurg 96, 569-575, 1993

Ringelstein EB, Koschorke S, Holling A, Thron A, Lambertz H, Minale C: Computed tomographic patterns of proven embolic brain infarctions. Ann Neurol 26, 759-765, 1989

Ringelstein EB, Weiller C: Hirninfarktmuster im Computertomogramm. Pathophysiologische Konzepte, Validierung und klinische Relevanz. Nervenarzt 61, 462-471, 1990

Sander D, Klingelhöfer J: Changes of circadian blood pressure patterns after hemodynamic and thromboembolic brain infarction. Stroke 25, 1730-1737, 1994

Sanfelippo MJ, Suberviola PD, Geimer NF: Development of a von Willebrand like syndrom after prolonged use of hydroxyethyl starch. Am J Clin Pathol 88, 653-655, 1987

Scandinavian stroke study group: Multicenter trial of hemodilution in acute ischemic stroke. Stroke 18, 691-699, 1987

Scandinavian stroke study group: Multicenter trial of hemodilution in acute ischemic stroke. Results of subgroup analyses. Stroke 19, 464-471, 1988

Seaman BVF, Engel R, Swank RL, Hissen W: Circadian periodicity in some physiological parameters of circulating blood. Nature 4999, 833-835, 1965

Second international study of infarct survival (ISIS-2): Randomised trial of intravenous streptokinase, oral aspirin, both or neither among 17187 cases of suspected acute myocardial infarction. Lancet II, 349-360, 1988

Sekhar LN, Wechsler LR, Yonas H, Luyckx K, Obrist W: Value of transcranial doppler examination in the diagnosis of cerebral vasospasm after subarachnoid hemorrhage. Neurosurgery 22, 813-821, 1988

Shoemaker WC, Appel PL, Waxman K, Schwartz S, Chang P: Clinical trial of survivors cardiorespiratory patterns as therapeutic goals in critically ill postoperative patients. Crit Care Med 10, 398-403, 1982

Shoemaker WC, Appel PL, Kram HB, Nathan RC, Thompson JL: Multicomponent noninvasive physiologic monitoring of circulatory function. Crit Care Med 16, 482-490, 1988

Shoemaker WC, Appel PL, Kram HB, Waxman K, Lee T-S: Prospective trial of supranormal values of survivors as therapeutic goals in high-risk surgical patients. Chest 94, 1176-1186, 1988

Shoemaker WC, Appel PL, Kram HB, Duarte D, Harrier HD, Ocampo HA: Comparison of hemodynamic and oxygen transport effects of dopamine and dobutamine in critically ill surgical patients. Chest 96, 120-126, 1989

Shoemaker WC, Kram HB: Effects of crystalloids and colloids on hemodynamics, oxygen transport and outcome in high-risk surgical patients. in: Simmons RC, Udekuo AS (eds) Debates in clinical surgery. Yearbook, Chicago 263-316, 1990

Shoemaker WC, Kram HB, Appel PL: Therapy of shock based on pathophysiology, monitoring, and oucome prediction. Crit Care Med 18, S19-S25, 1990

Shoemaker WC, Appel PL, Kram HB, Bishop MH, Abraham E: Temporal hemodynamic and oxygen transport patterns in medical patients with sepsis and septic shock. Chest 104, 1529-1536, 1993

Shoemaker WC, Appel PL, Kram HB, Bishop MH, Abraham E: Sequence of physiologic patterns in surgical septic shock. Crit Care Med 21, 1876-1889, 1993

Smith KE, Hachinski VC, Gibson CJ, Ciriello J: Changes in plasma catecholamine levels after insula damage in experimentel stroke. Brain Research 375, 182-185, 1986

Sommoggy S, Pfeiffer U, Sarmiento C: Perioperatives hämodynamisches Monitoring des aortofemoralen Bifurkationsbypasses: Pulmonalis-Einschwemmkatheter-Messung versus Impedanzcardiographie. Angio 4, 199-208, 1988

Staedt U: Hämorheologische, makro- und mikrozirkulatorische Parameter einschließlich ihrer Interaktionen bei Patienten mit akutem Hirninfarkt unter pathophysiologischen und therapeutischen Gesichtspunkten. Habilitationsschrift, Heidelberg, 1994

Stoll M, Hamann G, Jost V, Schimrigk K: Ein PC-gestütztes System zum Online-Monitoring von neurologischen Intensivpatienten. Biomed Technik 37, 37-41, 1992

Stoll M, Treib J, Seltmann A, Haaß A, Schimrigk K: Influence of hypervolemic therapy of acute stroke with low molecular weight hydroxyethyl starch on hemodynamics. Neurological Research 20, 231-234, 1998

Strand T, Asplund K, Eriksson S, Hägg E, Lithner F, Wester P-O: A randomized controlled trial of hemodilution therapy in acute ischemic stroke. Stroke 15, 980-989, 1984

Strand T: Evaluation of long-term outcome and safety after hemodilution therapy in acute ischemic stroke. Stroke 23, 657-662, 1992

Thomas DJ, Boulay GH, Marshall J, Pearson TC, Ross Russell RW, Symon L, Wetherley-Mein G, Zilkha E: Effect of haematocrit on cerebral blood-flow in man. Lancet II, 941-943, 1977

Thomas DJ: Whole blood viscosity and cerebral blood flow. Stroke 13, 285-287, 1982

Thorvaldsen P, Asplund K, Kuulasmaa K, Rajakangas A-M, Schroll M: Stroke incidence, case fatality, and mortality in the WHO MONICA Project. Stroke 26, 361-367, 1995

Tranmer BI, Gross CE, Kindt GW, Adey GR: Pulsatile versus nonpulsatile blood flow in the treatment of acute cerebral ischemia. Neurosurgery 19, 724-731, 1986

Tranmer BI, Keller TS, Kindt GW, Archer D: Loss of cerebral regulation during cardiac output variations in focal cerebral ischemia. J Neurosurg 77, 253-259, 1992

Treib J, Haaß A, Pindur G, Seyfert UT, Treib W, Grauer MT, Jung F, Wenzel E, Schimrigk K: HES 200/0,5 is not HES 200/0,5. Influence of the C2/C6 hydroxyethylation ratio of hydroxyethyl starch (HES) on hemorheology, coagulation and elimination kinetics. Thromb Haemost 74, 1452-1456, 1995

Treib J, Haaß A, Koch D, Stoll M, Ohlmann D, Schimrigk K: TCD-Untersuchung über den Einfluß der Hämodynamik auf die zerebrale Autoregulation beim akuten Hirninfarkt. Ultraschall in Med 17, 64-67, 1996

Treib J, Haaß A, Stoll M, Grauer MT: Monitoring and management of antihypertensive therapy induced deterioration in acute ischemic stroke. Am J Hypertens 9, 513-514, 1996

Treib J, Haaß A, Pindur G, Treib W, Wenzel E, Schimrigk K: Influence on intravascular molecular weight of hydroxyethyl starch on platelets during a long-term hemodilution. European Journal of Hematology 56, 168-172, 1996

Treib J, Haaß A, Pindur G, Grauer MT, Wenzel E, Schimrigk K: All medium starches are not the same: Influence of degree of substitution of hydroxyethyl starch on volumen effect, hemorheologic conditions and coagulation. Transfusion 36, 450-455, 1996

Treib J, Haaß A, Grauer MT, Stoll M, Koch D, Schimrigk K: Comparison of hypervolemic hemodilution concepts in acute stroke. Clinical Hemorheology 16, 367-375, 1996

Treib J, Haaß A, Krammer I, Stoll M, Grauer MT, Schimrigk K: Cardiac output in patients with acute stroke. Journal of Neurology 243, 575-578, 1996

Treib J, Haaß A, Stoll M, Grauer MT, Koch D, Ohlmann D, Schimrigk K: Influence of blood pressure and cardiac output on cerebral blood flow and autoregulation in acute stroke measured by TCD. European Journal of Neurology 3, 539-543, 1997

Treib J, Haaß A, Pindur G: Coagulation disorders caused by hydroxyethyl starch. Thrombosis and Haemostasis 78, 974-983, 1997

Treib J, Haaß A, Pindur G, Wenzel E, Schimrigk K: Blutungskomplikationen durch Hydroxyethylstärke sind vermeidbar. Deutsches Ärzteblatt 94, 2326-2330, 1997

Treib J, Haaß A: Rheologische Eigenschaften von Hydroxyethylstärke. Deutsche Medizinische Wochenschrift 122, 1319-1322, 1997

Treib J, Haaß A, Schmid-Schönbein H, Fröhlig G: Bedeutung der Hämodynamik beim akuten Hirninfarkt. Deutsches Ärzteblatt, 96, A-553-556, 1999

Treib J, Baron JF, Grauer MT, Strauss RG: An international view of hydroxyethyl starches. Intensive Care Medicine 25, 258-268, 1999

Treib J, Becker SC, Grauer MT, Haaß A: Transcraniel Doppler-monitoring of intracranial pressure therapy with mannitol, sorbitol and Glycerol in patients with acute stroke. European Neurology 40, 212-219, 1998

Treib J, Haaß A: Volumentherapie aus interdisziplinärer Sicht, Deutsches Ärzteblatt 96, 929-932, 1999

Treib J, Haaß A: Prävention des Hirninfarktes. Deutsches Ärzteblatt, in Druck

Vander Ark GD, Pomerantz M: Reversal of ischemic neurological signs by increasing the cardiac output. Surg Neurol 1, 257-258, 1979

Volc D, Schmidl F, Koch C: Hämodilution mit Dextran oder Hydoxyäthylstärke. Hämodynamische Veränderungen im transkraniellen Doppler-Monitoring. J Pharmacol u Ther 4, 11-16, 1995

Wannamethee G, Perry IJ, Shaper AG: Haematocrit, hypertension and risc of stroke. J Intern Med 235, 163-168, 1994

Warren JL, Bacon WE, Harris T, McBean AM, Foley DJ, Phillips C: The burden and outcomes associated with dehydration among US elderly, 1991. Am J Public Health 84, 1265-1269, 1994

Weber J, Heidelmeyer CF, Kubatz E, Brückner JB: Die Bestimmung des Herzzeitvolumens unter PEEP-Beatmung mit dem nichtinvasiven Bioimpedanzgerät "NCCOM 3" im Vergleich zur Thermodilutionsmethode. Anaesthesist 35, 744-747, 1986

Weinberg AD, Minaker KL: Dehydration, evaluation and management in older adults. JAMA 274, 1552-1556, 1995

Werner C, Hoffman WE, Baughman VL, Albrecht RF, am Esch JS: Effects of Sufentanil on cerebral blood flow, cerebral blood flow velocity, and metabolism in dogs. Anesth Analg 72, 177-181, 1991

Wityk RJ, Stern BJ: Ischemic stroke: Today and tomorrow. Crit Care Med 22, 1278-1293, 1994

Woo MA, Hamilton M, Stevenson LW, Vredevoe DL: Comparison of thermodilution and transthoracic electrical bioimpedance cardiac outputs. Heart Lung 20, 357-362, 1991

Wood JH, Snyder LL, Simeone FA: Failure of intravascular volume expansion without hemodilution to elevate cortical blood flow in region of experimental focal ischemia. J Neurosurg 56, 80-91, 1982

Wood JH, Simeone FA, Fink EA, Golden MA: Hypervolemic hemodilution in experimental cerebral ischemia. J Neurosurg 59, 500-509, 1983

Yamaguchi S, Kobayashi S, Yamashita K, Kitani M: Pial arterial pressure contribution to early ischemic brain edema. J Cereb Blood Flow Metab 9, 597-602, 1989

Yamauchi H, Fukuyama H, Ogawa M, Ouchi Y, Kimura J: Hemodilution improves cerebral hemodynamics in internal carotid artery occlusion. Stroke 24, 1885-1890, 1993

Yasaka M, Yamaguchi T, Oita J, Sawada T, Shichiri M, Omae T: Clinical features of recurrent embolization in acute cardioembolic stroke. Stroke 24, 1681-1685, 1993

del Zoppo GJ: Why do all drugs work in animals but none in stroke patients? Drug promoting cerebral blood flow. J Intern Med 237, 79-88, 1995

del Zoppo GJ: Acute Stroke. On the threshold of a therapy. N Engl J Med 333, 1632-1633, 1995

CHAPTER 2

Hetastarch for the Treatment
of Perioperative Hypotension

E. T. RILEY

Introduction

Rapid intravascular volume expansion is frequently required in the care of patients during surgery and in the intensive care unit. Crystalloid solutions (e.g. lactated Ringer's, normal saline, etc.) are used most frequently. In most cases, crystalloid solutions are adequate but not optimal [1]:

1. Crystalloid solutions rapidly redistribute throughout the extracellular fluid space. Since the body's intravascular space comprises 20% of the extracellular fluid space, only a fifth of the volume from an intravenous bolus of crystalloid solution will effectively expand blood volume.
2. The redistribution of the crystalloid into the extracellular fluid can increase edema. This can be problematic in major surgical cases or in patients in the intensive care unit.
3. Crystalloid solutions decrease the colloid oncotic pressure. This also exacerbates edema.

More suitable volume expanders would stay intravascular and not increase edema significantly. Alternatives to crystalloid solutions include blood products like packed red blood cells, fresh frozen plasma, and albumin. However, blood cells and fresh frozen plasma have substantial disease transmission risk associated with their use and should only be used to improve the oxygen carrying capacity of the patient's blood or to correct coagulation defects. There is no risk of disease transmission with albumin. However, the supply is limited and the cost is prohibitive.

The practical alternative are the artificial colloid solutions such as the gelatin solutions and the starch solutions. These solutions have no risk for disease transmission, can easily be supplied, and are reasonably priced. Following is a review of the use of hetastarch in anesthesia and the intensive care unit. Hetastarch is one of the more popular artificial colloids in use today.

Intravascular Fluid Volume, Colloid Oncotic Pressure, Edema

The main advantage of hetastarch over crystalloid solutions is that it stays intravascular. The half life of hetastarch is 9 ± 1 hours [2] and the effective duration of action is about 1 to 2 days [3]. The effective intravascular volume expansion is essentially equal to the amount infused. Ueyama et al. [4] used a dye dilution technique to measure a change in blood volume after volume loading. There was very close agreement between hetastarch volumes given and increases in blood volume (Fig. 1). Crystalloid solutions were not nearly as effective. Blood volume in this group only increased by about 1/4 of the amount of crystalloid given.

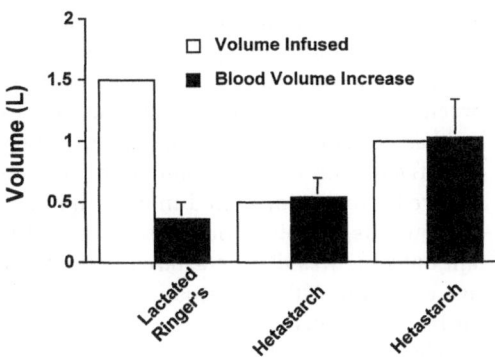

Fig. 1. Intravenous fluid loads of lactated Ringer's 1.5 L, hetastarch 0.5 L, or hetawomen prior to spinal anesthesia for Cesarean delivery. Data from Ueyama H, et al. Anesthesiology 1996, 85:A901 and personal communication with H. Ueyama, M.D.

The first advantage of hetastarch staying intravascular is that not as much needs to be given compared to crystalloid. Twice as much saline was required to maintain stable systemic and central pressures in a rabbit model of isovolemic hemodilution using hetastarch or saline [5]. This can be important during surgery or in the intensive care unit where fluid shifts or blood loss can be rapid and there is a need for rapid volume expansion.

The other important factor is that the use of hetastarch should decrease tissue edema compared to crystalloid solutions since more fluid stays intravascular and the colloid oncotic pressure is maintained. In patients having Whipple procedures it has been shown that volume replacement with hetastarch maintains colloid oncotic pressure whereas crystalloid volume replacement resulted in a significant decrease in colloid oncotic pressure [6]. Using another starch (dextran 70) Wennberg et al. found less fluid lung water compared to patients preloaded with crystalloid [7]. In an animal model (pigs made septic with *E. coli*), there was less edema in the animals resuscitated with hetastarch [8]. And in another animal model (hepatoenteric ischemia-reperfusion in rabbits), there was less tissue damage in animals treated with hetastarch compared to crystalloids [9].

Clinical Efficacy

There is substantial laboratory evidence and evidence from clinical measurements that hetastarch should be a better resuscitative fluid compared to crystalloid solutions. The question is whether these theoretical advantages translate to better clinical outcomes. The difficulty in answering this question is that when looking at ultimate outcomes (survival, days in the intensive care unit, Apgar scores, etc.) the type of fluid used for resuscitation will be only one of many factors affecting outcome. Of course, even a small improvement in such important outcomes as these are very significant. However, to show differences in these type of outcomes, prohibitively large data sets are needed. If one looks at surrogate outcomes (incidence of hypotension, amount of pressor drug needed to maintain blood pressure, etc.), the question then is are these significant enough to justify the added cost of using hetastarch. Following is a review of important clinical studies that demonstrate the clinical efficacy of hetastarch. This evidence is substantial, but not overwhelming. Whether this evidence is ample enough to justify the use of hetastarch in one's practice can only be determined by the individual practitioner.

One study that required few subjects to demonstrate a significant difference between hetastarch and crystalloid fluid for resuscitation was a study of patients who had had either coronary bypass or valve surgery. These patients were managed postoperatively with either crystalloid or hetastarch. As expected the crystalloid group required more fluid, gained more weight and the hetastarch group had higher cardiac outputs, systolic blood pressures, and lower hematocrits. However, the important outcome was that hetastarch patients spent significantly less time in the intensive care unit. Although this is not as important an outcome variable as survival, cardiac function, etc. a shortened intensive care unit stay does justify the added cost of using hetastarch [10].

Another cardiac surgery study also found shorter intensive care unit and hospital stays in the group of patients that received hetastarch volume loading. This was correlated with better perfusion of the gut mucosa (as measured by gut pH) and fewer post-operative complications [11]. In another cardiac surgery study, when acute plasmapheresis was used and the volume was replaced with either crystalloid or hetastarch, the hetastarch patients had a better outcome in terms of platelet count, colloid oncotic pressure, fibrinogen concentration, fluid balance, and blood loss [12].

Hetastarch is often used prior to spinal anesthesia to prevent hypotension from the sympathectomy that is invariably produced upon induction. In most comparisons between hetastarch and crystalloids the incidence of hypotension is reduced (Table 1). In addition to a lower incidence of hypotension, we found that the hypotension came on slower, it was less profound, required less treatment and heart rate was lower (Table 2) [13]. This makes for a smoother anesthetic that is easier to manage and may be more comfortable for the patient.

One area of anesthesia where fluid balance and tissue edema is crucial to outcome is in neurosurgery cases. In an experimental model on dogs Tranmer [14] found that crystalloid infusions increased intracranial pressure and decreased EEG power after a liquid nitrogen induced brain lesion. Hetastarch infusions had no effect on ICP and EEG power increased. Other laboratory studies have not been successful at showing that starch solutions decrease tissue edema associated with brain injury [5,15]. Unfortunately there are no clinical outcome studies of the effect of hetastarch on neurosurgery outcome. However, if the theoretical advantages of using colloids in

Table 1. The incidence of hypotension with spinal anesthesia with crystalloid and hetastarch preloads

Study	Population	Comparison	Hypotension crystalloid	Hypotension colloid	P
Sharma [28]	Post Partum Tubals	HES 500 mL LR 1 L	52%	16%	<0.05
Riley [13]	Cesarean	HES 500 mL + LR 1L LR 2 L	85%	45%	<0.05
Karinen [29]	Cesarean	HES 500 mL LR 1L	62%	38%	N.S.

HES = Hetastarch
X = 500 mL of Hartmann's solution

Table 2. Anesthetic block and hemodynamic variables from Riley et al. [13]

	Hetastarch	Lactated Ringer's
Baseline SBP (mm Hg)	117 ± 13	116 ±15
Baseline heart rate (bpm)	81 ± 10	84 ±12
Minimum SBP (mm Hg)ᵃ	93 ± 12	85 ± 12*
Maximum heart rate (bpm)ᵃ	104 ± 16	115 ± 17*
% Patients with hypotension	45%	85%*
Supplemental ephedrine (mg)	7 ± 9	12 ± 14
Doses of ephedrineᵇ	0 (0–6)	2 (0–10)*
Time to hypotension (min)	10 ± 7	7 ± 4*

Mean ± S.D.
* P <0.05
ᵃ Before any supplemental ephedrine administration
ᵇ Median number (range) of supplemental 5 mg doses of ephedrine given for hypotension

neurosurgery hold true, there would seem to be good reason to expect improved outcome with the use of hetastarch over crystalloid in neurosurgery.

Hetastarch: Complications and Other Colloids

Comparisons of hetastarch with other colloids seldom shows any clinically significant differences [5,15–18]. Given that the effect on colloid pressure and volume expansion should be very similar, this is expected. Any clinically significant differences between colloids would relate to side effects. Hetastarch has relatively few adverse side effects. The most serious is an association with anaphylactoid or anaphylactic reactions [19]. This can manifest itself as anything from a skin rash to severe bronchospasm and hypotension. Fortunately the incidence of these reactions is low (lower than reactions to gelatin and dextran) [20]. The only colloid available with a lower incidence of allergic reactions is albumin. In a study of 750 patients that received hetastarch, no significant reactions occurred [21]. In my clinical practice at Stanford, I have not had any reactions more significant than skin rashes and mild wheezing. This suggests that allergic reactions to hetastarch are rare.

The adverse effect of hetastarch on coagulation has been well documented [22]. It is caused by an interference with the factor VIII/vonWillebrand complex. This effect can be limited by using Hetastarch solutions with a lower *in vivo* molecular weight [23]. Currently in the U.S. the hetastarch that is available has a high *in vivo* molecular weight. In order to avoid any affect on coagulation I limit hetastarch to 1 liter in an adult patient. This is very conservative and bigger doses are probably safe. Claes et al. [24] found no difference in coagulation in neurosurgical and gynecological patients that had had volume replacement with hetastarch or albumin except for a decrease in the acute phase reaction of factor VIII coagulant and von Willebrand factor (which contributes to post-operative hypercoagulability). When compared to a gelatin colloid solution, average doses of 2500 mls of hetastarch given to orthopedic patients had no significant effect on coagulation [25]. In intensive care unit patients the use of albumin vs. hetastarch had no affect on coagulation parameters despite average use of 4 liters over 5 days [26]. In contrast, cardiac surgery patients given hetastarch right after bypass had a trend towards increased bleeding compared to patients that did not receive hetastarch or only got hetastarch postoperatively [27]. This suggests there are certain high risk situations (e.g. immediately post bypass) where it is inadvisable to use hetastarch.

Summary

There is substantial laboratory and clinical evidence that hetastarch is an effective volume replacement product. Because it tends to stay intravascular and not be distributed to the extracellular fluid space, compared to crystalloids, it causes less edema and is a more effective volume replacement. How much of an effect this has on outcome is probably small, but significant enough to justify its use in higher risk cases. Significant side effects are rare.

References

1. Gorin NC, Najman A, Duhamel G: Autologous bone marrow transplantation in acute myelocytic leukemia. *The Lancet* 8020: 1050, 197711. Griffel MI, Kaufman BS: Pharmacology of colloids and crystalloids. Crit Care Clin 1992; 8: 23553
2. Behne M, Thomas H, Bremerich DH, Lischke V, Asskali F, Forster H: The pharmacokinetics of acetyl starch as a plasma volume expander in patients undergoing elective surgery. Anesth Analg 1998; 86: 856–60
3. Smiley LE: The use of hetastarch for plasma expansion. Probl Vet Med 1992; 4: 652–67
4. Ueyama H, Yan-Ling H, Tanigami H, Mashimo T, Yoshiya I: The effects of crystalloid and colloid preload on the blood volume in the parturient undergoing spinal anesthesia for elective Cesarean section. Anesthesiology 1996; 85: A901
5. Zornow MH, Scheller MS, Todd MM, Moore SS: Acute cerebral effects of isotonic crystalloid and colloid solutions following cryogenic brain injury in the rabbit. Anesthesiology 1988; 69: 180–4
6. Prien T, Backhaus N, Pelster F, Pircher W, Bunte H, Lawin P: Effect of intraoperative fluid administration and colloid osmotic pressure on the formation of intestinal edema during gastrointestinal surgery. J Clin Anesth 1990; 2: 317–23
7. Wennberg E, Frid I, Haljamae H: Comparison of Ringer's acetate with 3% dextran 70 for volume loading before extradural caesarean section. Br J Anaesth 1990; 65: 654–60
8. Baum TD, Wang H, Rothschild HR, Gang DL, Fink MP: Mesenteric oxygen metabolism, ileal mucosal hydrogen ion concentration, and tissue edema after crystalloid or colloid resuscitation in porcine endotoxic shock: comparison of Ringer's lactate and 6% hetastarch. Circ Shock 1990; 30: 385–97
9. Nielsen VG, Tan S, Brix AE, Baird MS, Parks DA: Hextend (hetastarch solution) decreases multiple organ injury and xanthine oxidase release after hepatoenteric ischemia-reperfusion in rabbits. Crit Care Med 1997; 25: 1565–74
10. Ley SJ, Miller K, Skov P, Preisig P: Crystalloid versus colloid fluid therapy after cardiac surgery. Heart Lung 1990; 19: 31–40
11. Mythen MG, Webb AR: Perioperative plasma volume expansion reduces the incidence of gut mucosal hypoperfusion during cardiac surgery. Arch Surg 1995; 130: 423–9
12. Boldt J, Kling D, Zickmann B, Jacobi M, von Bormann B, Dapper F, Hempelmann G: Acute plasmapheresis during cardiac surgery: volume replacement by crystalloids versus colloids. J Cardiothorac Anesth 1990; 4: 564–70
13. Riley ET, Cohen SE, Rubenstein AJ, Flanagan B: Prevention of hypotension after spinal anesthesia for cesarean section: six percent hetastarch versus lactated Ringer's solution [see comments]. Anesth Analg 1995; 81: 838–42

14. Tranmer BI, Iacobacci RI, Kindt GW: Effects of crystalloid and colloid infusions on intracranial pressure and computerized electroencephalographic data in dogs with vasogenic brain edema [see comments]. Neurosurgery 1989; 25: 173–8; discussion 8–9

15. Goulin GD, Duthie SE, Zornow MH, Scheller MS, Peterson BM: Global cerebral ischemia: effects of pentastarch after reperfusion [see comments]. Anesth Analg 1994; 79: 1036–42

16. Aly Hassan A, Lochbuehler H, Frey L, Messmer K: Global tissue oxygenation during normovolaemic haemodilution in young children. Paediatr Anaesth 1997; 7: 197–204

17. Belcher P, Lennox SC: Avoidance of blood transfusion in coronary artery surgery: a trial of hydroxyethyl starch. Ann Thorac Surg 1984; 37: 365–70

18. Baron JF, De Kegel D, Prost AC, Mundler O, Arthaud M, Basset G, Maistre G, Masson F, Carayon A, Landault C, et al.: Low molecular weight hydroxyethyl starch 6% compared to albumin 4% during intentional hemodilution. Intensive Care Med 1991; 17: 141–8

19. Cullen MJ, Singer M: Severe anaphylactoid reaction to hydroxyethyl starch. Anaesthesia 1990; 45: 1041–2

20. Dieterich HJ, Kraft D, Sirtl C, Laubenthal H, Schimetta W, Polz W, Gerlach E, Peter K: Hydroxyethyl starch antibodies in humans: incidence and clinical relevance. Anesth Analg 1998; 86: 1123–6

21. Bothner U, Georgieff M, Vogt NH: Assessment of the safety and tolerance of 6% hydroxyethyl starch (200/0.5) solution: a randomized, controlled epidemiology study. Anesth Analg 1998; 86: 850–5

22. Treib J, Haass A: Hydroxyethyl starch [letter; comment]. J Neurosurg 1997; 86: 574–5

23. Treib J, Haass A, Pindur G, Grauer MT, Jung F, Wenzel E, Schimrigk K: Increased haemorrhagic risk after repeated infusion of highly substituted medium molecular weight hydroxyethyl starch. Arzneimittelforschung 1997; 47: 18–22

24. Claes Y, Van Hemelrijck J, Van Gerven M, Arnout J, Vermylen J, Weidler B, Van Aken H: Influence of hydroxyethyl starch on coagulation in patients during the perioperative period. Anesth Analg 1992; 75: 24–30

25. Beyer R, Harmening U, Rittmeyer O, Zielmann S, Mielck F, Kazmaier S, Kettler D: Use of modified fluid gelatin and hydroxyethyl starch for colloidal volume replacement in major orthopaedic surgery. Br J Anaesth 1997; 78: 44–50

26. Boldt J, Heesen M, Muller M, Pabsdorf M, Hempelmann G: The effects of albumin versus hydroxyethyl starch solution on cardiorespiratory and circulatory variables in critically ill patients [see comments]. Anesth Analg 1996; 83: 254–61

27. Cope JT, Banks D, Mauney MC, Lucktong T, Shockey KS, Kron IL, Tribble CG: Intraoperative hetastarch infusion impairs hemostasis after cardiac operations. Ann Thorac Surg 1997; 63: 78–82; discussion –3

28. Sharma SK, Gajraj NM, Sidawi JE: Prevention of hypotension during spinal anesthesia: a comparison of intravascular administration of hetastarch versus lactated Ringer's solution. Anesth Analg 1997; 84: 111–4

29. Karinen J, Rasanen J, Alahuhta S, Jouppila R, Jouppila P: Effect of crystalloid and colloid preloading on uteroplacental and maternal haemodynamic state during spinal anaesthesia for caesarean section. Br J Anaesth 1995; 75: 531–5

CHAPTER 3

Volume Therapy and Ocular Diseases

V. SCHERER, K. W. RUPRECHT

Introduction

The precise etiology of ocular vascular occlusions is not known in all details. The pathogenesis may be associated with abnormalities of blood rheology and coagulation. Frequently, it is associated with an underlying systemic disease (Table 1). Despite many years of investigation and research, some principles of the pathophysiology and therapy of this disease entity remain unclear.

Ocular vascular occlusions usually occur suddenly and present a dramatic visual loss, but there are also chronic and intermediate forms.

Due to the absence of a causal therapy of ocular microcirculation disorders and because of their heterogenous nature, a common treatment standard has not yet been established. Besides minimizing the risk profile for atherosclerosis or any different underlying disease, one of the most effective therapeutic approaches may be volume therapy.

Basically, the following ocular vascular diseases are associated with a substantial circulation disorder and, due to their pathogenesis, seem to be eligible for hemodilution:

1. Venous occlusive disease of the retina
2. Arterial obstructive disease of the retina
3. Noninflammatory ischemic optic neuropathy

Venous Occlusive Disease of the Retina

The acute occlusion of the central retinal vein or its branches is mostly a result of both local and systemic factors. The clinical picture may be roughly divided into those conditions that produce a retinal ischemia, while patients are usually aware of a sudden and painless decrease in visual acuity and those with a much milder progression regarding appearance, symptoms, and course. The occlusion may affect the central retinal vein (CRVO) or just retinal vein branches.

Table 1. Relevant risk factors for ocular blood flow [4]

Atherosclerosis
Elevated intraocular pressure
Arterial hypertension
Focal vasospasm
Vasculitis
Nicotine
Drug-induced blood pressure reduction
Anatomic variants

Table 2. Indication and contraindication for volume therapy of venous occlusive diseases of the retina [2, 6]

Indications	
Symptoms	<8 wks
Hematocrit	≥39%
Platelets	450×109/l
Age	<80 y
Heart	No cardiovascular contraindications
Contraindications	
Absolute	Global decompensated heart failure
	Severe coagulopathy
	Renal failure (creatinine >2 mg/dl)
Relative	Renal failure (creatinine between 1.2 and 2.0 mg/dl)
	Arterial hypertension (systole >170 mm Hg)

Main complications of central retinal vein occlusions are:
1. The formation of a macular edema and consequently a significant visual loss
2. The development of a secondary glaucoma due to neovascularization following retinal ischemia

The actual pathophysiological mechanism producing the typical findings is not entirely understood. For the development of CRVO, either a physical blockage at the level of the lamina cribrosa or hemodynamic factors resulting in an obstruction of blood flow may be responsible. Most patients present with both conditions.

Because the etiology of venous occlusive diseases of the retina is not known in all details, no "golden" treatment standard has been established so far. Many different treatment approaches have been subject of clinical trials: aspirin, plasmapheresis, pentoxifylline, steroids, rheologic drugs, hyperbaric oxygen (HBO-therapy), urokinase, streptokinase, drug-induced vasodilatation, cryotherapy of the ciliary body, retinal laser treatment, carbogen inhalation, etc.

The most important part of the therapeutic regimen is to analyze the overall risk profile and minimize possible adverse factors. First-line treatment is volume therapy according to a standard pattern depending on the patient's health status (Table 2). Controlled clinical trials could demonstrate the effectiveness of either isovolemic or hypervolemic hemodilution[1, 2, 5] (Table 3).

Arterial Obstructive Disease of the Eye

Arterial obstruction of the retinal vessels is one of the most dramatic events seen by the ophthalmologist [4] and represents an emergency situation.

Retinal artery obstruction occurs mostly at either the level of the optic nerve head or close to an arterial bifurcation. It is characterized by an initial opacification of the affected, ischemic retina segment as a result of an edema.

Predominantly, patients present with a sudden, painless loss of vision. The clinical picture is typically striking. Depending on the localization of the occlusion and the dimension of the affected retina, the patient may notice a visual field defect or loss of visual acuity, or both.

Table 3. Volume therapy of venous occlusive disease of the retina [2, 6]

	Hematocrit	Dosage
I. Inpatient treatment (10 days): optimal hematocrit range between 33% and 37%		
Stable cardiovascular status	>45%	500 ml HES + 500 ml Phlebotomy
	40%–45%	250 ml HES + 250 ml Phlebotomy
	<40%	250 ml HES
Minor cardiac insufficiency	>40%	250 ml HES + 250 ml Phlebotomy
	<40%	250 ml HES
II. Outpatient treatment (4–5 wks): optimal hematocrit range between 33% and 37%	>39%	250 ml HES + 250 ml Phlebotomy

The etiology of retinal artery obstruction in most of the cases remains unclear. In some cases, an association with a systemic disorder could be found (Table 4).

Treatment results are generally unsatisfactory and disappointing. Some patients recover good visual acuity following a central retinal artery obstruction with no treatment, while others may reestablish normal blood flow and visual acuity several days after treatment [4].

The most relevant factor for treatment success is the period of time in which a total lack of blood flow (ischemia) to the inner retina can be tolerated. After this

Table 4. Major systemic and topical conditions associated with arterial obstructive disease [4]

Systemic conditions	
Embolus formation [4]	Carotid artery disease
	Atherosclerosis
	Cardiac or valvular disease
	Myocardial infarction (mural thrombus)
	Tumors, etc.
Coagulopathies [3]	Oral contraceptives
	Platelet and factor abnormalities
	Sickle cell disease
	Homocysteinemia etc.
Miscellaneous [3]	Giant cell arteritis
	Polyarteritis nodosa
	Systemic lupus erythematosus
	Diabetes mellitus etc.
Topical conditions	
Injury [2]	Compression
	Penetrating injury
	Retrobulbar injection, etc.
Increased intraocular pressure	
Miscellaneous [2]	Optic nerve drusen
	Optic neuritis
	Toxocara canis infection, etc.

Table 5. Treatment of central retinal artery occlusion [3, 6]

Latency between first symptoms and beginning of treatment not more than 12 h
    Immediate treatment: hydroxyethyl starch (HES), massage of the eyeball, catheter-mediated
    lysis (depending on the underlying systemic diseases)
    Long-term treatment: aspirin (100 mg/d), for weeks, heparinization (depending on the risk
    profile)

Special treatment is required for inflammatory diseases of ocular vessels.
    Latency between first symptoms and beginning of treatment between 12 h and 2 d
    Immediate treatment: isovolemic hemodilution for 10 d
    Long-term treatment: aspirin (100 mg/d)

Similar treatment is recommended for branch retinal artery occlusions.

lapse time of total obstruction, changes are irreversible and the patient suffers permanent visual loss. Therefore, immediate treatment is required:

The therapeutic goal is always to restore the retinal blood flow as soon as possible. Lowering the intraocular pressure is one of the methods of immediate treatment, e.g., by local or systemic drugs, ocular massage, or. rarely. by paracentesis. Different concepts such as gas inhalation, pharmacologic vasodilatation, hyperbaric oxygen therapy, or even acupuncture have been subjects of discussion. Another effective treatment is local or systemic fibrinolysis, e.g., by urokinase, if the symptom-to-treatment-interval is small enough.

Moreover, sufficient intravascular fluid for maintaining stable hemodynamics is essential for therapeutic success. Volume therapy appears to be one of the few effective concepts to reduce retinal ischemia.

The objective of volume therapy is to optimize blood flow by lowering hematocrit (by values between 38% and 40%). It must be considered that diminishing the number of blood cells means a reduction of oxygen carriers. Treatment planning and realization should be carried out in cooperation with the internist (Table 5).

In the long run, minimization of the general risk profile for atherosclerosis, determination of the underlying etiology, and keeping intravascular conditions stable should be the goal of treatment. Depending on the underlying disease, additional drug therapy with aspirin, pentoxifylline, or steroids may be helpful.

Noninflammatory Anterior Ischemic Optic Neuropathy

As risk factors and pathogenesis are, in many patients, similar to retinal artery obstruction, treatment possibilities are also limited. Volume therapy may be one weapon in the rather small therapeutic arsenal (Table 6).

Table 6. Treatment of noninflammatory anterior ischemic optic neuropathy (time interval between first symptoms and treatment ≤10 days)

Immediate treatment:	Isovolemic hemodilution for 10 d
Long-term treatment:	Aspirin (100 mg/d)

Table 7. Therapeutic success of volume therapy according to the literature [6]

	Volume therapy	Spontaneous course
Venous obstructive disease of the retina: increase in visual acuity	37%–53%	5%–20%
Arterial obstructive disease of the retina: increase in visual acuity	0%–50%	<10%
Noninflammatory anterior ischemic optic neuropathy: increase vs. loss in visual acuity	32%–45% vs. 0%–19%	0%–24% vs. 11%–25%

Summary (Table 7)

1. Venous occlusive disease of the retina: the positive effect of volume therapy on visual acuity could be demonstrated in controlled clinical trials for both, ischemic and nonischemic retinal vein occlusion.
2. Arterial obstructive disease of the retina: a reliable efficiency of volume therapy for the treatment of central or branch retinal artery obstruction has not been proven in controlled trials. Generally, the results of treatment of central retinal artery occlusion are unsatisfactory. In the absence of causal therapy, volume therapy offers a small chance of improving visual function, particularly for patients who do not qualify for fibrinolysis due to cardiovascular problems or lapse of time.
3. Anterior ischemic optic neuropathy (AION): particularly patients with decreased retinal function may benefit if treatment starts within the first days after visual loss. The reliable effectiveness of volume therapy for AION has not been proven in controlled clinical trials.

Hence, volume therapy represents an important tool in the management of vascular eye diseases. Decisive for its success are mechanism, site and degree of microcirculation disorder, and, moreover, the time interval between onset of symptoms and initial therapy.

References

1. Dhalluin JF, Glacet-Bernard A, Lelong F, Coscas G, Soubrane G (1998) Traitement par hémodilutionisovolémique des occlusions de la veine centrale de la rétine récentes. Ophtalmologie 12: 442–445
2. Hansen LL (1994) Treatment possibilities of central retinal vein occlusion. Ophthalmologe 91:131–45
3. Krause A (1995) Arterielle Gefäßverschlüsse in der Netzhaut und im Nervus opticus. In: Kampik A, Grehn F (eds) Durchblutungsstörungen am Auge. Bücherei der Augenarztes. Enke-Verlag, Stuttgart, pp 92–96
4. Sanborn GE, Magargal LE (1998) Arterial obstructive disease of the eye. In: Duane's Ophthalmology on CD-ROM. Lippincott-Raven Publishers, Hagerstown
5. Wiek J (1995) Hämodilution bei okulärer Durchblutungsstörung. In: Kampik A, Grehn F (eds) Durchblutungsstörungen am Auge. Bücherei des Augenarztes. Enke-Verlag, Stuttgart, pp 97–103
6. Wolf S, Arend O, Bertram B, Remky A, Schulte K, Wald KJ, Reim M (1994) Hemodilution therapy in central retinal vein occlusion. One-year results of a prospective randomized study. Graefes Arch Clin Exp Ophthalmol 232:33–39

CHAPTER 4

Volume Therapy in the Field of Otolaryngology, Head and Neck Surgery

F. WALDFAHRER, H. IRO

Introduction

When volume therapy is applied in otorhinolaryngology and head and neck surgery, it is mainly used in the sense of rheologic therapy to improve microcirculation and not chiefly to substitute volume. Three important groups of indications for rheologic therapy must be distinguished:
1. Acute cochleovestibular failure
2. Acquired peripheral palsy of the facial nerve
3. Increasing the perfusion of microvascular flaps

Rheologic Therapy in Acute Cochleovestibular Failure

The term "acute cochleovestibular failure" summarizes sudden sensorineural hearing loss, acute tinnitus with or without sensorineural hearing loss, and acute failure of the peripheral vestibular organ. The annual incidence is estimated to be five to 20 cases per 100,000 [8, 14]. It is very important to distinguish clearly between symptomatic and idiopathic cochleovestibular disorders. For example, noise exposure, acoustic traumas with high peaks of noise and pressure, blunt injuries, tumors of the cerebellopontine angle, and encephalomyelitis disseminata can cause symptomatic acute hearing loss, tinnitus and/or dizziness.

As the term "idiopathic" suggests, the causes of acute sensorineural hearing loss still remain unclear. It is suspected that either viral infections or autoimmune reactions are causally related to this disease. Vascular compromise is also under discussion [1, 3, 8, 11, 12, 14, 16]. All three of these possible causes of sudden, idiopathic sensorineural hearing loss can bring about an alteration of the cochlear microcirculation. As a consequence, rheologic therapy is applied empirically in order to improve microcirculation of the cochleovestibular apparatus [3, 5, 9].

Acute tinnitus and acute vestibular failure are suspected as having the same pathophysiological background and, therefore, are treated in a similar way [6, 16, 17].

In the past, dextrans were widely used for this purpose; but the high rates of adverse effects, especially anaphylactic and allergic reactions and the need for "priming" have raised the demand for alternative drugs. Hydroxyethyl starch (HES) not only has been demonstrated to be superior to dextran in therapeutic efficacy but also has fewer adverse effects [5, 14]. Today, HES must be considered the drug of choice in rheologic therapy of acute cochleovestibular disorders [5, 14].

Therapy with HES is usually used in combination with other rheologic drugs, such as pentoxifylline or naftidrofuryl. Recently, pentoxifylline was identified as an inhibitor of tumor necrosis alpha factor, an important factor in the inflammation cascade. Additionally, corticosteroids have antiinflammatory and antiedematous properties and are frequently coadministered. Steroids were the only group of drugs which proved to be effective in monotherapy of sudden sensorineural hearing loss [14]. Lidocaine can be applied as a tinnitus-depressant drug with cochlear and central targets [17].

Table 1 depicts the infusion scheme currently used by the authors for patients with acute cochleovestibular disorders with reference to the suggested etiopathology. This 10-day schedule is applied exclusively under in-patient conditions.

The authors reviewed the records of 305 patients with acute cochleovestibular disorders treated within 12 months at the Department of Otorhinolaryngology, Head and Neck Surgery, Saarland University Hospital, Germany.

A slight male preponderance (57%) was recognized; the mean age at presentation was 45.8 ± 16.5 years. Twenty two per cent reported a similar event in the past and 20% had undergone some kind of rheologic treatment before admission. All patients underwent rheologic infusion therapy as described in Table 1; when tinnitus was absent, no lidocaine was administered. In patients with mild hearing loss, usually no prednisolone was given.

Two hundred four patients (67%) complained of hearing loss, 204 suffered from tinnitus, and 97 (32%) had dizziness and balance disorders (Fig. 1).

Table 1. Therapy of acute cochleovestibular disorders: current scheme in use of the Department of Otorhinolaryngology, Head and Neck Surgery, Saarland University

Time	Dosage	Route of administration
Days 1–2	250 ml HES 10% 200/0.4	IV
	Pentoxifylline 300 mg in Ringer solution	IV
	Pentoxifylline 400 mg	Orally every 8 h
Days 3–4	Pentoxifylline 300 mg in Ringer solution	IV
	Pentoxifylline 400 mg	Orally every 8 h
	10 ml Lidocaine[a] 2% in physiologic saline solution	IV
Days 5–6	Pentoxifylline 300 mg in Ringer solution	IV
	Pentoxifylline 400 mg	Orally every 8 h
	12 ml Lidocaine[a] 2% in physiologic saline solution	IV
Days 7–8	Pentoxifylline 300 mg in Ringer solution	IV
	Pentoxifylline 400 mg	Orally every 8 h
	14 ml Lidocaine[a] 2% in physiologic saline solution	IV
Days 9–10	Pentoxifylline 300 mg in Ringer solution	IV
	Pentoxifylline 400 mg	Orally every 8 h
	16 ml Lidocaine[a] 2% in physiologic saline solution	IV

[a] Lidocaine is only administered in the presence of tinnitus. Usually prednisolone is coadministered beginning with 250 mg IV on day 1. On the following days, dosage is reduced in 50 mg steps to 100 mg on day 4. With day 5, prednisolone is given orally and reduced in 20 mg steps.

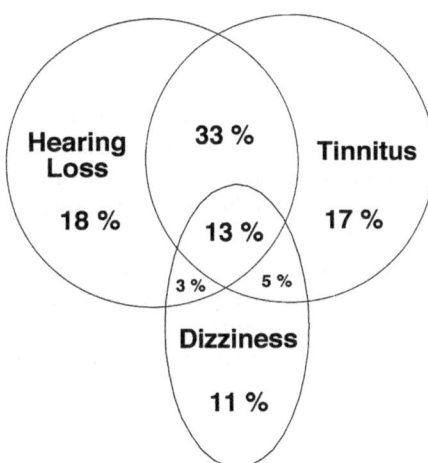

Fig. 1. Symptoms in 305 patients with
acute cochleovestibular disorders

Pure tone audiometry detected hearing loss in the low frequency band in 11%, in the middle frequency band in 7%, in the high frequency band in 33%, and a pantonal hearing loss in 30% of the patients with hearing impairment. Nineteen per cent had combined hearing loss. Forty two per cent had a moderate degree of hearing loss (according to Jerger's categorization), 18% a mild degree, and 27% a severe degree. In 13%, a profound hearing loss was detected.

In 91.1% of the patients, the therapeutic schedule was fulfilled completely; in 3.9%, the dosage of pentoxifylline or lidocaine had to be reduced because of adverse side effects; and, in 3%, the therapy was canceled prematurely on the patients' demands. Adverse side effects included hypertension (6.9%), headache (4.3%), dizziness (1.3%), nausea (5.9%), and cardiovascular side effects such as palpations, arrhythmia, or heart pain (5.9%). In 9.2%, administration of an additional drug was necessary due to adverse effects. In 6.2%, the symptoms disappeared spontaneously without further interventions.

Eighty eight per cent of the patients with hearing loss recognized a improvement of hearing after a maximum of 10 days of treatment; 45% already felt relief after 3 days . In pure tone audiometry, 80% of the patients showed significant recovery. The presence or absence of tinnitus or dizziness seemed to be of no prognostic relevance, as statistic assessment demonstrated. Also, age, gender, degree of hearing loss, and the presence of cardiovascular risk factors could not be identified as prognostic factors, as other authors had shown [3, 10, 14]. On the other hand, the interval between appearance of symptoms and start of treatment was demonstrated to be a significant prognostic factor. While 86% of the patients treated within 3 days after the onset of hearing loss showed audiometric improvement, only 27% of those treated more than 2 weeks after onset of hearing loss experienced hearing recovery. When treatment started between the 4th and the 7th days or between the 8th and the 14th days after the onset of symptoms, audiometric improvements were detected in 65% and 35%, respectively.

Sixty seven per cent of the patients with tinnitus felt noticeable relief within the 10 days of infusion therapy.

One half of the patients who demonstrated signs of complete unilateral vestibular failure showed normal caloric responses after rheologic treatment. However, 50% of the patients had persisting unilateral vestibular failure with signs of central vestiblar compensation. Therefore, it is to be concluded that acute vestibular failure is not always irreversible, as proposed by some authors.

Summarizing our results, rheologic infusion therapy was shown to be highly effective and, in general, well-tolerated. Although the influence of spontaneous remissions on the results cannot be calculated [12, 22], rheologic infusion therapy should be instituted immediately in cases of acute cochleovestibular disorders. But, even if a complete recovery is achieved, patients should be re-examined carefully using audiometric tests and imaging procedures, because we detected vestibular schwannomas by MRI in two patients with sudden sensorineural hearing loss and good response to rheologic infusion therapy.

Rheologic Therapy in Acquired Peripheral Palsy of the Facial Nerve

Palsies of the seventh cranial nerve are divided into central forms, with intact innervation of the frontal branch, and peripheral forms, including palsy of the frontal branch. This chapter deals only with peripheral palsies, since central palsies of the facial nerve are the neurologist's responsibility. Table 2 summarizes common causes of peripheral facial palsy.

As a consequence of detection of *Borrelia burgdorferi* and Herpes simplex virus as two important infectious agents causative for acute facial palsy, today, only 35% of acute facial palsies remain "idiopathic" in comparison to 100% 20 years ago.

However, it is suspected that occult reactivation of a herpes simplex virus infection is also responsible for a large amount of today's "idiopathic" palsies [4, 15]. In some cases, hints of an autoimmune disease can be detected.

All patients with acute facial palsy must be examined very carefully, using otomicroscopy, pure tone audiometry, electromyography and -neurography, and imaging of the temporal bone and the cerebellopontine angle. Serology is performed to detect Borrelia burgdorferi, HSV, and VZV as causative infectious agents. Facial palsy is classified according to the House facial nerve grading system [13].

Therapy of acute facial palsy is orientated towards etiopathology whenever possible. Middle ear disease, neoplasms, and injuries with immediate palsy of the facial nerve should be treated preferentially by surgery, including reconstruction of the fa-

Table 2. Common causes of acquired peripheral palsy of the facial nerve [modified according to 4, 13, 15, 19]

Trauma:	temporal bone fractures, penetrating wounds
Middle ear disease:	cholesteatoma, acute otitis media, acute mastoiditis
Infections:	Herpes simplex, Varicella zoster (Ramsay Hunt syndrome), Borrelia burgdorferi (Lyme disease)
Neoplasia:	carcinoma of parotid gland or temporal bone, facial neurinoma, meningioma, paraganglioma
Syndromes:	Melkersson-Rosenthal, Guillain-Barre
"Idiopathic":	Bell's palsy

Table 3. Rheologic infusion therapy of acute peripheral facial palsy used at the Department of Otorhinolaryngology, Head and Neck Surgery, Saarland University (modified after Stennert)

Time	Dosage	Route of administration
Days 1–10	500 ml HES 6% 200/0,4	IV
	Pentoxifylline 300 mg	
	in Ringer solution	IV
	Pentoxifylline 400 mg	Oral every 8 h
Day 1	Prednisolone 250 mg	IV
Day 2	Prednisolone 200 mg	IV
Day 3	Prednisolone 150 mg	IV
Days 4–5	Prednisolone 100 mg	IV
Days 6–7	Prednisolone 80 mg	Oral
Day 8	Prednisolone 60 mg	Oral
Day 9	Prednisolone 40 mg	Oral
Day 10	Prednisolone 20 mg	Oral

cial nerve, if necessary. In Lyme disease, an antibiotic treatment, usually with third generation cephelosporine, must be applied. Herpes virus infections are commonly treated with antiviral agents such as aciclovir, famciclovir, or valaciclovir.

In facial palsy cases of uncertain origin, an initial treatment with antibiotic and virustatic agents should be considered until serologic tests have excluded Lyme disease and reactivation of herpes virus as causes. In our hospital, every patient with facial palsy of uncertain origin is initially treated with aciclovir and ceftriaxone.

Rheologic infusion therapy in facial palsy was introduced by the German otolaryngologist E. Stennert in 1979 [18] and consisted of administration of corticosteroids, dextrans, and pentoxifylline. Today, dextran has been replaced by hydroxyethyl starch (HES). In our department, we use a modified Stennert scheme as depicted in Table 3.

This scheme is applied (in addition to antiviral and/or antibacterial agents), in all cases of infectious facial palsy, in cases of delayed facial palsy after temporal bone injuries, and in all cases of "idiopathic" facial palsy. Adverse side effects include hypertension, hyperglycemia, nausea, and headache. Up to now, we have not observed one case of persisting pruritus [7], but we always inform our patients about this possible adverse side effect of HES in the applied total dose of 300 g.

Rheologic Therapy to Increase the Perfusion of Microvascular Flaps

Free flaps with microvascular anastomoses are widely used in otorhinolaryngology, head and neck surgery for reconstruction of defects especially after resection of large tumors. Table 4 enumerates the most commonly applied microvascular flaps.

The success of head and neck reconstruction using microvascular free flaps is strongly related to proper perfusion of the flap through its anastomosed arterial and venous vessels. Impairment of macro- and microcirculation due to thromboembolic ischemia or arterial spasms jeopardizes the survival of the flap. Therefore, rheologic therapy is applied to increase perfusion and microcirculation in order to ensure the survival of the flap. In our department, we use high-dose pentoxifylline (100 mg/h via perfusor) together with hydroxyethyl starch (HES 10%, 200/0.5, 250 ml/day), start-

Table 4. Microvascular free soft tissue flaps and visceral flaps for head and neck reconstruction [2, 20, 21]

Flap	Arterial vessel(s)
Radial forearm flap	A. radialis
Lateral arm flap	A. profunda brachii, A. collateralis radialis
Lateral thigh flap	A. profunda femoris and perforators
Rectus abdominalis flap	A. epigastrica superior profunda, A. epigastrica inferior profunda
Latissimus dorsi flap	A. thoracodorsalis
Jejunum flap	A. mesenterica
Omentum flap	A. gastroepiploica dextra

ing before the vessels are anastomosed. Although this particular application of rheologic therapy has not been evaluated under scientific conditions (prospective randomized studies) until now, from the empiric point of view it seems to be effective. However, a few patients do not tolerate these high pentoxifylline doses; in these cases the dose is reduced to 75 mg/h or 50 mg/h. We recommend this kind of rheologic therapy in all cases of "critical" flap perfusion.

Acknowledgements. The authors wish to thank Ms. Christine Bindel for reviewing the records of 305 patients undergoing rheologic infusion therapy and analyzing the data very conscientiously.

References

1. Baloh RW (1998) Dizziness, hearing loss, and tinnitus. F.A. Davis, Philadelphia
2. Bootz F, Müller GH (1992) Mikrovaskuläre Gewebetransplantation im Kopf-Hals-Bereich. Georg Thieme Verlag, Stuttgart
3. Byl FM (1984) Sudden hearing loss: eight years' experience and suggested prognostic table. Laryngoscope 94:647–661
4. Coker NJ, Vrabec JT (1998) Acute paralysis of the facial nerve. In: Bailey BJ, Calhoun KH (eds) Head and neck surgery – otolaryngology. Lippincott-Raven, Philadelphia, New York, second edition, pp 2107–2124
5. Desloovere C, Meyer-Breiting E, v Ilberg C (1988) Randomisierte Doppelblindstudie zur Hörsturztherapie: Erste Ergebnisse. HNO 36:417–422
6. Feldmann H (1998) Tinnitus. Georg Thieme Verlag, Stuttgart, second edition
7. Gall H, Kaufmann R, v Ehr M, Schumann K, Sterry W (1993) Persistierender Pruritus nach Hydroxyethylstärke-Infusionen. Hautarzt 44:713–716
8. Hashisaki GT (1998) Sudden sensory hearing loss. In: Bailey BJ, Calhoun KH (eds) (1998) Head and neck surgery – otolaryngology. Lippincott-Raven, Philadelphia, New York, second edition, pp 2192–2198
9. Laskawi R, Schrader B, Schröder M, Poser R, v d Brelie R (1987) Zur Therapie des Hörsturzes – Naftidrofuryl (Dusodril) und Pentoxifyllin (Trental) im Vergleich. Laryng Rhinol Otol 66:242–245
10. Linssen O, Schultz-Coulon HJ (1997) Prognostische Kriterien beim Hörsturz. HNO 45: 22–29
11. McCabe BF (1979) Autoimmune sensorineural hearing loss. Ann Otol 88:585–589
12. Mattox DE, Simmons FB (1977) Natural history of sudden sensorineural hearing loss. Ann Otol Rhinol Laryngol 86:463–480
13. May M (1986) The facial nerve. Georg Thieme Verlag, New York, Stuttgart
14. Michel O (1994) Der Hörsturz. Georg Thieme Verlag, Stuttgart
15. Peitersen E (1992) Natural history of Bell's palsy. Acta Otolaryngol Suppl 492:122–124
16. Sataloff RT, Sataloff J (1993) Hearing loss. Marcel Dekker, New York, Basel, Hong Kong, third edition

17. Shulman A; Aran JM, Tonndorf J, Feldmann H, Vernon JA (1997) Tinnitus diagnosis/treatment. Singular Publishing Group, San Diego, London
18. Stennert E (1979) Bell's palsy – a new concept of treatment. Arch Oto-Rhino-Laryngol 225:265–268
19. Stennert E: Fazialisparesen. In: Helms J, Naumann HH, Herberhold C, Kastenbauer ER (eds) (1994) Oto-Rhino-Laryngologie in Klinik und Praxis. Band 1 Ohr. Georg Thieme Verlag, Stuttgart, pp 666–701
20. Strauch B, Vasconez LO, Hall-Findlay EJ (eds) (1998) Grabb's Encyclopedia of flaps. Head and neck. Lippincott-Raven, Philadelphia, New York, second edition
21. Urken ML, Cheney ML, Sullivan MJ, Biller HF (1995) Atlas of regional and free flaps for head and neck reconstruction. Raven Press, New York
22. Weinaug P (1984) Die Spontanremission beim Hörsturz: HNO 32:346–351

CHAPTER 5

Volume Therapy in Neurosurgery

F. CORTBUS, W. I. STEUDEL

Introduction

Hypervolemic therapy today plays an important role in neurosurgical intensive care, particularly
1. in the treatment of reduced cerebral perfusion pressure (CPP) following severe head injury and
2. in the treatment of cerebral vasospasm following subarachnoid hemorrhage.

Therefore, both these aspects of neurosurgical hypervolemic therapy are to be described in more detail.

Severe Head Injury

In the management of patients with severe head injury, there has long been an appreciation of substantially restricting intravenous fluids. This was based on the fear of increased oedema formation with a generous supply of fluids and resulting symptoms of herniation.

With the introduction by Lundberg in the mid-1960s [1] of intracranial pressure (ICP) monitoring to clinical neurosurgical practice, interest in obtaining ICP measurements in patients with severe head injuries grew. In 1977, Miller et al. [2] showed the adverse effect of raised ICP on outcome of head injury and provided the first estimation of the frequency of intracranial hypertension in a consecutive series of comatose patients, including both patients with intracranial hematomas and those with diffuse brain injury. Since then, neurosurgical management strategies for patients with severe head injuries have focussed on reducing elevated ICP.

After the studies of Zwetnow and others [3, 4], it has been accepted that the CPP can be derived from the difference between mean arterial pressure (MAP) and ICP:

CPP=MAP−ICP

Since that time, the monitoring of arterial and intracranial pressures has become more widespread in intensive care units. However, treatment strategies, tended to emphasize the institution of therapy at certain threshold levels of increased ICP. Michael Rosner and others [5, 6] during the 1980s have been the strongest advocates of basing treatment strategies of head-injured patients more directly on influencing the CPP rather than exclusively on decreasing elevated ICP.

At the beginning of the 1990s, the research team surrounding Douglas Miller succeeded to prove in a study of 124 patients [7] that periods of CPP below 60 mm Hg for up to 5 min occurred in approximately 75% of patients in intensive care with

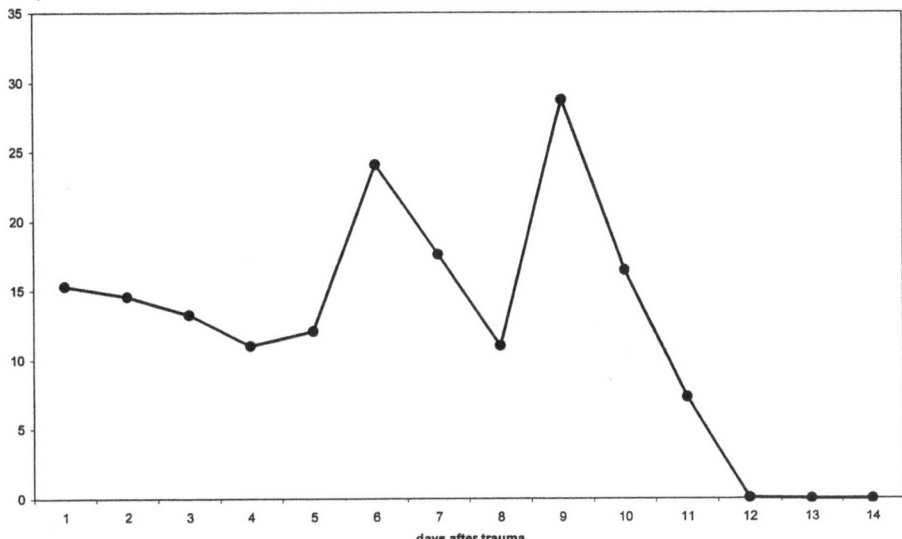

Fig. 1. Percentage of monitoring time per day that CPP reductions under 60 mm Hg were observed in 60 patients after head injury

varying degrees of head injury. Collection of these data was possible via multimodal, computerized monitoring in which the key variables were collected at 1 min intervals. Research on them was able to show clearly and significantly that such episodes of reduced CPP negatively influenced the outcome of traumatic brain injury.

In further examinations of the same group [8], it was shown in a consecutive series of 74 patients that brain injury patients in intensive care spend up to 29% of monitoring time with CPP below 60 mm Hg, although they are monitored every minute with a multimodal monitoring device. The interesting factor here is the distribution of the episodes of reduced CPP, which shows pronounced peaks at day 5 and day 9, after a slight initial decrease (Fig. 1).

On examination of the effects of arterial hypotension, increased ICP, and the combination of the two on episodes of reduced CPP, it could be observed, especially initially and in the late phases after trauma, that arterial hypotension (defined as a MAP under 80 mm Hg) was present for up to 78% of the period of reduced CPP (Fig. 2). This gives a very good impression of severity of the arterial hypotension problem in managing head injuries, even under the best intensive care with minute-by-minute monitoring of key variables.

After statistical analysis of the data of this study [8], a strong and significant correlation between systemic arterial hypotension, CPP, and bad outcome in brain-injured patients was found. Changes in cerebral perfusion lie at the root of this. In a hypotensive patient, even minor increases in ICP can lead to substantial deterioration of cerebral perfusion and therefore cause secondary ischemia. On the other hand, elevated blood pressure in a patient with high ICP can protect that patient from cerebral ischemia.

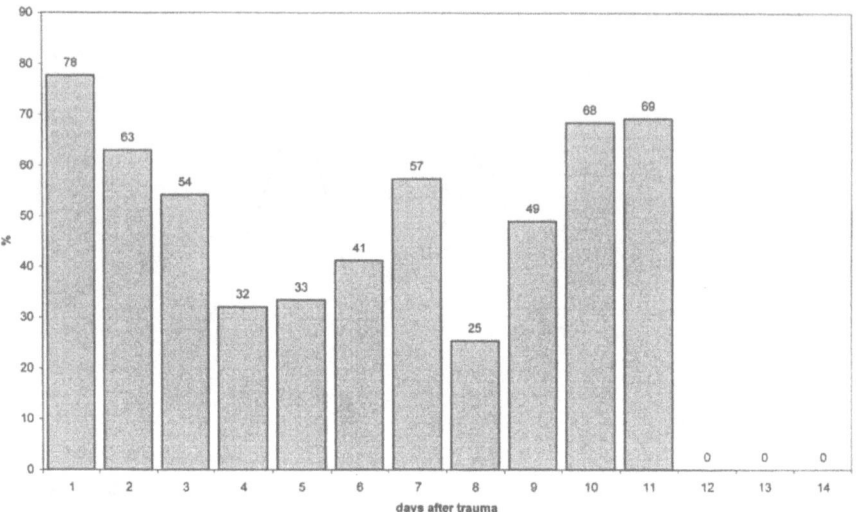

Fig. 2. Presence of arterial hypotension (MAP <80 mmHg) during periods of reduced CPP under 60 mmHg in percent of CPP reduction time in 60 patients after head injury

The detrimental effect of systemic hypotension in the preclinical period was also very impressively shown in the data analysis of the Traumatic Coma Data Bank [9]. In this prospective study carried out by five large American trauma centers, a singular observation of preclinical hypotension (systolic blood pressure below 90 mm Hg) led to a doubling of mortality (Table 1).

As a consequence of these research findings, sufficient volume therapy of supplying electrolytic solutions and plasma expanders to optimate the CPP has been favoured since the beginning of the 1980s.

This altered therapy strategy has been entered into the Guidelines for the Management of Severe Head Injury [10] presented in 1996 in the *Journal of Neurotrauma* after critical analysis of all literature published on brain injury since 1966. The recommendations contained in these guidelines concerning preclinical and clinical volume therapy along with fast restoration of stable blood circulation and arterial pressure above 90 mm Hg were basically taken over by the American Brain Injury Consortium (ABIC) and the European Brain Injury Consortium- (EBIC).

The management of CPP after brain injury is based principally on achieving a positive balance of about 600–1000 ml, regarding the perspiratio insensibilis, as well as the maintenance of a central venous pressure of 10–12 mm Hg. Additionally, cat-

Table 1. Effect of preclinical systemic hypotension on mortality after severe head injury

	Patients (n)	Mortality
No hypotension	456	27%
With hypotension	113	60%

echolamines are applied when volume-loading alone is insufficient for reaching a CPP of at least 70 mm Hg [11].

The effect of an artificial increase in blood pressure by volume therapy and catecholamines on the ICP has been systematically examined in patients with brain injury. Bouma and Muizelaar [12] as well as Bruce et al. [13] found only slight increases of ICP of up to 4 mm Hg by artificially increasing the mean arterial pressure from 90 mm Hg to 120 mm Hg. However, in many cases, there were also decreases in ICP. Inducing arterial hypertension via volume therapy and catecholamines seems to be a viable route to take in order to improve cerebral perfusion.

More recent studies in which the CPP was kept as planned above 70 mm Hg [11, 14, 15] report a median mortality of 21% in patients with severe brain injury with a Glasgow Coma Scale score ranging from 3 to 7 points. This is a substantial decrease from the 40% mortality rate attained from data of the American Traumatic Coma Data Bank [16] for patients with the same Glasgow Coma Scale score.

Thus, on the whole, the change over the past 30 years from restriction of fluids to today's widespread volume therapy with an increase in arterial blood pressure and CPP has led to clear improvement in the outcome of patients with severe brain injuries.

Subarachnoid Hemorrhage

The concept of cerebral vasospasm after subarachnoid hemorrhage was introduced by Ecker and Riemenschneider [17]. They showed that a reduction of the caliber of basal arteries seen on second cerebral angiograms is very common and may lead to an ischemic deficit or a manifested ischemic insult. Clinically, the vasospasm becomes symptomatic as delayed ischemic neurological deficit (DIND) through an impairment of vigilance, a paresis, or aphasia. The arterial narrowing leads to an increase in blood velocity which can be measured by transcranial Doppler ultrasound (Table 2).

Reviewing all the literature of the past 30 years [18], a vasospasm could be detected angiographically in 43.28% of 31,168 patients after subarachnoid hemorrhage. In 32.28% of the patients, DIND occurred after subarachnoid hemorrhage. In a therapeutically uninfluenced course, patients suffering from clinical vasospasm with DIND showed a complete recovery in 35.7% of cases, a permanent neurological deficit in 34.0%, and a lethal outcome in 30.3%.

Thus, vasospasm is the most frequent cause of death and handicap following subarachnoid hemorrhage. Progress in intensive care of patients with clinical vasospasm is seen as primarily responsible for the reduction in mortality from more than 40% in the 1960s to approximately 8% at the beginning of the 1990s [39].

Table 2. Interpretation of transcranial Doppler for vasospasm

Mean MCA velocity in cm/s	MCA/ICA ratio	Interpretation
< 120	<3	Normal
120–200	3–6	Mild vasospasm
>200	>6	Severe vasospasm

Numerous studies have been performed on the prevention and treatment of vasospasm. Nimodipine, rtPA, Tirilazad, and endothelin antagonists are the drugs that have been tested. In addition, transluminous angioplasty and hyperdynamic therapy also must be mentioned. Concerning therapy strategies using medication, existing studies have not produced any significant, unequivocal results. With Nimodipine alone, a considerable number of studies show a tendency towards improved outcome without, however, being capable of significantly influencing statistically angiographic vasospasm or mortality. Tirilazad and other more recent medications have not been able to fulfill the initially high expectations.

Only hyperdynamic therapy, also called triple-H therapy, consisting of hypervolemia, hemodilution, and induced hypertension has established itself. In 1976, Kosnik and Hunt first reported the value of induced hypertension for reducing deficits caused by vasospasm. A short time afterwards, Pritz et al. [20] reported on the usefulness of intravascular volume expansion. Also, in further clinical series [21, 22], the practice of increasing arterial blood pressure through volume expansion and catecholamines could also be confirmed.

After subarachnoid hemorrhage, patients tend towards hypovolemia in the early clinical course [23–25, 30], often in connection with constant hypotonic phases. However, for a large percentage these hypotonic phases lead to ischemic deficits and should therefore be avoided. The starting of hyperdynamic therapy [26, 27, 32] prophylactically, before the vasospasm has been manifested angiographically, clinically, or with Doppler sonography can also greatly contribute to a reduction in ischemic deficits caused by vasospasm.

Objectives of hyperdynamic therapy or prophylaxis (Table 3) recognized today are principally:

1. Hypervolemia, when a CVP of 10–12 cm H_2O or a
   pulmonary-capillary wedge pressure of 14 mm Hg is aimed for.
2. Hemodilution, in which a hematocrit of 30% is considered optimal [31].
3. Induced hypertension, ideally with systolic blood pressure of up to 200 mm
   Hg or MAPs of 100–130 mm Hg.

During practical application of triple-H therapy, electrolyte solutions and plasma expanders are used in order to achieve hypervolemia. In so doing, an intravenous supply of at least 3000 ml of fluid per day is aimed for. In prophylactic volume expansion, many centers apply two thirds electrolyte solutions and one third colloid solutions, whereas in therapeutic volume expansion two thirds of colloids are infused.

In the United States, the use of hydroxyethyl starch (HES) is looked at rather critically, due to the necessity of therapy lasting several days and to risks of disturbances in the coagulation system [28, 29]. In this context, there are reports on coagulopathies with intracerebral bleeding. In patients with impaired kidney function and increased retention values, therapy with HES is connected to the risk of oliguric kidney failure

Table 3. Endpoints of hyperdynamic therapy

Hypovolemia	Hemodilution	Induced hypertension
CVP = 10–12 cm H_2O	Hkt = 30%	Systolic BP ≤ 200 mm Hg
PCWP = 14 mm Hg		MAP = 100–130 mm Hg

[33-35] due to the substantial storage of the substance in the reticuloendothelial system. In these cases, close monitoring of retention values is therefore indispensible. All studies reporting on coagulation disorders after HES administration have used Hetastarch, a high molecular weight (MW) hydroxyethyl starch with a MW of 450,000 to 480,000 D and a long-lasting volume effect. This starch leads to a large increase in partial thromboplastin time and to an 80% drop in the factor VIII/von Willebrand factor complex [40, 41].

More recent studies [42, 43] indicate that through the administration of HES with a low in vivo MW, coagulation disorders can be avoided. Unfortunately, these starches are not available everywhere in the world [44]. In Germany, 18 different kinds of HES are commercially available and in use. Eleven of them have medium MW (200 kDa) and three have low MW (70 kDa). The application of various kinds of HES up to a volume of 1500 ml/day is therefore more widespread in German-speaking countries.

However, in many neurosurgical centers, the use of fluid gelatine has been approved. In a series of 120,000 units of 4% modified liquid gelatine, no side effects due to dosage had occurred. In particular, there was no impairment of surgical hemostasis or kidney function, although more than 1,000 patients received more than 2,000 ml in a space of 24 h.

In order to attain sufficient arterial blood pressure, additional catecholamines may be required. This can be achieved by a dopamine infusion starting with 4 µg/kg per minute. If the arterial blood pressure is still insufficient, with a dopamine infusion rate of 14-16 µg/kg per minute, switching to norepinephrine with a starting dose of 0.02 µg/kg/min is recommended to avoid severe tachycardia, the most common side effect of high dopamine doses. Of course, extensive monitoring, including invasive arterial blood pressure measurement are required in such an invasive haemodynamic therapy (Table 4).

Therapeutic influence and prevention of ischemic deficits in hyperdynamic therapy are achieved by optimizing the hemodynamic and the patient's rheologic status. By increasing the mean arterial pressure, cerebral perfusion pressure can be improved. Volume expansion enhances the supply of potentially ischemic brain areas through dilatation of the leptomeningeal collaterals. A decrease in hematocrit reduces the viscosity of the blood and thus lowers cerebrovascular resistance, by which the cerebral blood flow (CBF) is vastly improved.

If this hyperdynamic therapy is applied in patients with clinical vasospasm and delayed neurological deficit after subarachnoid hemorrhage, remission of the deficit can be achieved in 62% of the patients [18]. In 38% of the cases, hyperdynamic therapy

Table 4. Hyperdynamic therapy

Hypovolemia	
Electrolyte solutions	1000 mm-3000 mm
Colloids	
HES	3× 250 ml-3×500 ml
Fluid gelatin	3×250 ml-5×500 ml
Hemodilution (see above)	
Induced hypertension	
Dopamine	4-10 µg/kg per minute
Norepinephrine	0.02-0.2 µg/kg per minute

is not successful. The mortality rate in the group of patients who had been treated unsuccessfully is 46%.

In total, there have been 73 studies in the past 30 years on the outcome of patients under hyperdynamic therapy for a DIND, reporting on 2111 patients in all. Of these, 54% showed a good recovery under hyperdynamic therapy, 28.5% recovered with a permanent deficit, and 17.5% died. This is a considerable improvement in outcome, compared to the natural course of patients with DIND portrayed at the beginning.

If, however, one merely looks at more recent studies, a further improvement in outcome is noticeable, with a decrease of mortality after subarachnoid hemorrhage down to approximately 8%. This reduction of mortality and morbidity using hyperdynamic therapy has by now become the main argument for early operative care of ruptured aneurysms, as the massive increase of hemorrheological parameters can only be applied without increased danger of secondary hemorrhage in clipped aneurysms.

Conclusion

In the treatment of patients with severe brain injury, a complete change has taken place in the past 30 years, from traditional fluid restriction to adequate volume resuscitation with maintenance of sufficient cerebral perfusion pressure. Hypervolemic therapy in combination with induced hypertension has proved to be a safe and efficient method of improving outcome in patients with severe head injury.

In treating clinical vasospasm with DIND after subarachnoid hemorrhage, hemodilution, hypervolemia, and induced hypertension are nowadays the international standard. Here, too, a significant improvement in outcome is noticeable.

References

1. Lundberg NJ, Troupp H, Lorin H (1965) Continuous recording of the ventricular fluid pressure in patients with severe acute traumatic brain injury. J Neurosurg 22:581–590
2. Miller JD, Becker DP, Ward JD, et al (1977) Significance of intracranial hypertension in severe head injury. J Neurosurg 47:508–516
3. Zwetnow N (1970) Effects of increased cerebrospinal fluid pressure on the blood flow and on the energy metabolism of the brain. Acta Physiol Scand 339:1–31
4. Miller J D, Stanek AE, Langfitt TW (1982) Concepts of cerebral perfusion pressure and vascular compression during intracranial hypertension. In: ? (eds) Cerebral blood flow. Elsevier, Amsterdam, pp 411–432 (Progress in brain research, vol 35)
5. Rosner M J, Coley I (1986) Cerebral perfusion pressure, intracranial pressure, and head elevation. J Neurosurg 65:636–641
6. Rosner MJ, Coley I (1987) Cerebral perfusion pressure: a hemodynamic mechanism of mannitol and the postmannitol hemogram. J Neurosurg 21:147–156
7. Jones PA, Andrews PJD, Midgley S, et al (1994) Measuring the burden of secondary insults in head-injured patients during intensive care. J Neurosurg Anesth 6:4–14
8. Cortbus F, Jones PA, Miller JD, et al (1994) Cause, distribution, and significance of episodes of reduced cerebral perfusion pressure. Acta Neurochir (Wien) 130:117–124
9. Chesnut RM, Marshall LF, Klauber MR, et al (1993) The role of secondary brain injury in determining outcome of severe head injury. J Trauma 34:216–222

10. Bullock MR, Povlishock JT (1996) Guidelines for the management of severe head injury J Neurotrauma 13:641–794
11. Rosner MJ, Daughton S (1990) Cerebral perfusion pressure management of head injury. J Trauma 30:933–941
12. Bouma GJ, Muizelaar JP (1990) Relationship between cardiac output and cerebral blood flow in patients with intact and with impaired autoregulation. J Neurosurg 73:368–374
13. Bruce DA, Langfitt TW, Miller JD, et al (1973) Regional cerebral blood flow, intracranial pressure, and brain metabolism in comatose patients. J Neurosurg 38:131–144
14. Fortune JB, Feustel, PJ, Weigle CGM, et al (1994) Continuous measurement of jugular venous oxygen saturation in response to transient elevations of blood pressure in head-injured patients. J Neurosurg 80:461–468
15. Yoshida A, Shima T, Okada Y, et al (1993) Outcome of patients with severe head injury. Evaluation by cerebral perfusion pressure. In: Nakamura N, Hashimoto T, Yasue M (eds) Recent advances in neurotraumatology. Springer, Berlin Heidelberg New York, pp 309–312
16. Marshall LF, Gautille T, Klauber MR (1991) The outcome of severe closed head injury J Neurosurg 75:36–38
17. Ecker A, Riemenschneider PA (1951) Arteriographic demonstration of spasm of the intracranial arteries: with special reference to saccular aneurysms. J Neurosurg 8:600–607
18. Dorsch N, King MT (1994) A review of cerebral vasospasm in aneurysmal subarachnoid hemorrhage. J Clin Neurosci 1:19–26
19. Kosnik EJ, Hunt WE (1976) Postoperative hypertension in the management of patients with intracranial arterial aneurysms. J Neurosurg 45:148–154
20. Pritz MB, Giannotta SL, Kindt GW, et al (1978) Treatment of patients with neurological deficits associated with cerebral vasospasm by intravascular volume expansion. J Neurosurg 3:364–368
21. Kassell NF, Peerless SJ, Durward QJ, et al (1982) Treatment of ischemic deficits from vasospasm with intravascular volume expansion and induced arterial hypertension. Neurosurgery 11:337–343
22. Awad IA, Carter LP, Spetzler RF, et al (1987) Clinical vasospasm after subarachnoid hemorrhage: response to hypervolemic hemodilution and arterial hypertension. Stroke 18:365–372
23. Wijdicks EFM, Vermeulen M, Hijdra A, et al (1985) Hyponatremia and cerebral infarction in patients with ruptured intracranial aneurysma: is fluid restriction harmful? Ann Neurol 17:137–140
24. Maroon JC, Nelson PB (1979) Hypovolemia in patients with subarachnoid hemorrhage: treatment implications. Neurosurgery 4:223–226
25. Wijdicks EFM, Vermeulen M, t Haaf JA, et al (1985) Volume depletion and natriuresis in patients with ruptured intracranial aneurysms. Ann Neurol 18:211–216
26. Solomon RA, Fink ME, Lennihan L (1988) Prophylactic volume expansion therapy for the prevention of delayed cerebral ischemia after early aneurysm surgery. Arch Neurol 45:325–332
27. Solomon RA, Fink ME, Lennihan L (1988) Early aneurysm surgery and prophylactic hypervolemic hypertensive therapy for the treatment of aneurysmal subarachnoid hemorrhage. Neurosurgery 23:699–704
28. Bianchine JR (1987) Intracranial bleeding during treatment with hydroxyethyl starch. Letter in reply. New Engl J Med 317:965
29. Trumble ER, Muizelaar JP, Myseros JS (1995) Coagulopathy with the use of hetastarch in the treatment of vasospasm J Neurosurg 82:44–47
30. Kudo T, Suzuki S Iwabuchi T (1981) Importance of monitoring the circulating blood volume in patients with cerebral vasospasm after subarachnoid hemorrhage. Neurosurgery 9:514–520
31. Muizelaar JP, Becker DP (1986) Induced hypertension for the treatment of cerebral ischemia after subarachnoid hemorrhage. Direct effect on cerebral blood flow. Surg Neurol 25:317–325
32. Origitano TC, Wascher TM, Reichmann OH, Anderson DE (1990) Sustained increased cerebral blood flow with prophylactic hypertensive hypervolemic hemodilution ("triple-H" therapy) after subarachnoid hemorrhage. Neurosurgery 27:729–740
33. Dehne MG, Muhling J, Sablotzki A, et al (1997) Effect of hydroxyethyl starch solutions on kidney function in surgical intensive care patients. Anästhesiol Intensivmed Notfallmed 32:348–354
34. Waldhausen P, Kiesewetter H, Leipnitz G, et al (1991) Hydroxyethyl starch-induced transient renal failure in pre-existing glomerular damage. Acta Med Austriaca 18 [Suppl 1]:52–55
35. Ginz HF, Gottschall V, Schwarzkopf G, Walter K (1998) Excessive tissue storage of colloids in the reticuloendothelial system. Anaesthesist 47:330–334

36. Lundsgaard-Hansen P, Tschirren B (1980) Clinical experience with 120,000 units of modified fluid gelatin. Dev Biol Stand 48:251–256
37. Barker FG, Ogilvy CS (1996) Efficacy of prophylactic nimodipine for delayed ischemic deficit after subarachnoid hemorrhage: a meta-analysis. J Neurosurg 84:405–414
38. Allen GS, Ahn HS, Preziosi TJ, et al (1983) Cerebral arterial spasm – a controlled trial of nimodipine in patients with subarachnoid hemorrhage. N Engl J Med 308:619–624
39. Kassell NF, Shaffey ME, Shaffey CI (1992) Cerebral vasospasm following aneurysmal subarachnoid hemorrhage. In: Apuzzo MLJ (ed) Brain surgery, complication avoidance, and management. Churchill Livingstone, New York, pp 847–856
40. Treib J, Haass (1997) Hydroxyethyl starch. J Neurosurg 86:574–575
41. Treib J, Haass A, Pindur G, et al (1995) HES 2000.5 is not HES 2000.5. Influence of the C2/C6 hydroxyethylation ratio of hydroxyethyl starch (HES) on haemorrheology, coagulation, and elimination kinetics. Thromb Haemost 74:1452–1456
42. Treib J, Haass A, Pindur G et al (1996) All medium starches are not the same: influence of degree of hydroxyethyl substitution of hydroxyethyl starch on plasma volume, haemorrheologic conditions, and coagulation. Transfusion 36:450–455
43. Treib J, Haass A, Pindur G (1997) Coagulation disorders caused by hydroxyethyl starch. Thromb Haemost 78:974–983
44. Muizelaar JP (1996) Response (letter to the editor). J Neurosurg 85:368

Crystalloids or Colloids for Volume Replacement in Anesthesia and Intensive Care Medicine?

J. BOLDT

Introduction

Adequate volume therapy is a mainstay for managing patients in the perioperative period. Absolute or relative blood volume deficits often occur during surgery and in the postoperative period. Aside from apparent blood loss, fluid deficits can occur in the absence of obvious fluid loss secondary to generalized alterations of the endothelial barrier resulting in diffuse capillary leak. Hypovolemia is associated with flow alterations which are inadequate to fulfill the nutritive role of the circulation. During this hypovolemia-related low output syndrome (LOS), the organism tries to compensate for perfusion deficits by redistribution of flow to vital organs (e.g., heart and brain), resulting in an underperfusion of other organs such as gut, kidneys, muscles, and skin. Various inflammatory mediators and circulating vasoactive substances are of particular importance for impaired perfusion in this situation. Activation of the sympathetic nervous system and the renin-angiotensin system (RAS) are compensatory mechanisms to maintain peripheral perfusion. Although this compensatory neurohumoral activation is beneficial at first, this mechanism becomes deleterious and may be involved in the bad outcome of the critically ill.

Fluid administration restores plasma volume and increases venous return to the heart, thus increasing cardiac output and improving systemic hemodynamics and organ perfusion. Shoemaker and coworkers [1] and Boyd et al. [2] have demonstrated the importance to maintain VO_2 and DO_2 at high levels to reduce the incidence of multiple organ failure (MOF) and overall mortality in high-risk surgical patients.

Three aspects are of major importance when volume replacement is considered:

1. The type of fluid must be decided.
2. The amount of fluid must be defined.
3. The criteria for guiding volume therapy must be defined.

The inherent risk of transmission of viral and immunological diseases has forced us to reduce the use of allogeneic blood and blood products. There is an ongoing controversy whether crystalloids or colloids should be infused for volume replacement [3–9]. Large volumes of crystalloids, which are necessary for effectively increasing plasma volume, may be associated with marked hemodilution and subsequent reduction in colloid osmotic pressure (COP), followed by the risk of increasing interstitial edema and an impaired organ function (e.g., pulmonary function). Colloids have been established for rapid restoration of the circulating plasma volume, thus avoiding excessive fluid accumulation, particularly in the interstitial tissue. The crystalloid/colloid debate has been widened in recent years to a colloid/colloid debate, since colloids have proven to be of benefit for volume therapy in these patients [10].

The primary goal of volume administration is to guarantee stable systemic hemodynamics. An important aspect for fluid therapy in this situation is the avoidance of interstitial edema. Tissue edema is related to an imbalance in the sum of the Starling forces across capillary membranes or an increase in protein permeability, by which an increase in fluid flux in the interstitial space is promoted. A decrease in membrane integrity, an increase in hydrostatic pressure, and a decrease in intravascular colloid oncotic pressure will induce a fluid movement across the microvascular membrane and produce interstitial fluid accumulation.

Possibilities of Volume Replacement in the Perioperative Period

Several solutions for volume replacement are available, varying with regard to their physicochemical and volume-expanding properties.

Allogenic blood and blood products should be avoided as far as possible because of their potential risk of transmitting infectious diseases. Patients with impaired hemostasis often needed fresh frozen plasma (FFP) or platelet concentrations. Careful attention is necessary to evaluate the oxygen-carrying capacity of the patients. It has to be taken into account that limitations of cardiac and pulmonary insufficiencies will influence the components of oxygen delivery.

Crystalloids can be subdivided into hypotonic (e.g., dextrose in water), isotonic (e.g., lactated Ringer's solution), and hypertonic solutions (e.g., 7.5% saline solution, mannitol). The underlying electrolyte status of the patient must be kept in mind when selecting the fluid for volume replacement (Table 1). Crystalloids are freely permeable to the vascular membrane and therefore distributed in the plasma and interstitial fluid volume. After 1,000 ml of saline infusion, plasma volume was expanded by only 180 ml [11]. As anticipated by several studies, approximately 25% of the infused saline remained in the intravascular compartment and 75% had extravasated into the interstitium [12]. Crystalloid solutions will lower plasma osmolality and drive water into the interstitial space. Thus, large volumes of crystalloids are required for restoring sufficient hemodynamics. Crystalloid solutions have to be given in a four- to fivefold amount, compared to colloids, to exert similar circulatory effects [13]. When infusing such high quantities of unbuffered saline, hyperchloremic acidosis theoretically could complicate this type of fluid therapy. Additionally, dilution of plasma protein concentration is accompanied by a (critical) reduction in plasma colloid oncotic pressure.

The naturally occurring plasma protein widely used for volume replacement is albumin . It is generally held to be safe and the kind of solution by which patients would profit most. The molecular weight (MW) of albumin ranges from 66,000 to 69,000 dalton. Due to its preparation procedures, it is free from risk of transmitting

Table 1. Examples of volume necessary to expand plasma volume by 1000 ml (mod. from [9])

	Increased PV (ml)	Infused volume (ml)	Increased IFV (ml)	Increased ICV (ml)
5% Albumin	1000	1000		
25% Albumin	1000	250	−750	
5% Dextrose	1000	14,000	3700	9,300
RL	1000	4700	3700	

PV plasma volume; IFV interstitial fluid volume; ICV intracellular volume; RL lactated Ringer's solution infections. 5% albumin is iso-oncotic, whereas 20% or 25% solution is markedly hyperoncotic, so that total plasma volume is expanded by translocation of fluid from the interstitial to the intravascular compartment. The effects of 5% albumin are not well-predictable: infusion of 500 ml of albumin expanded plasma volume by 490 ml or 750 ml. The retention of the infused albumin in the intravascular compartment, and therefore its hemodynamic efficacy, greatly vary with regard to the patient's disease. In patients with altered vascular endothelial integrity, albumin may pass into the interstitial space, by which fluid shift from the intravascular compartment is promoted. Dextran is a synthetic colloid not used very often in Europe. Dextrans are linear polysaccharide molecules of high MW (HMW). Two different preparations are available: 6% dextran 70 (average MW 70,000 dalton) and 10% dextran 40 (average MW 40,000 dalton). Increase of plasma volume after infusion of 1,000 ml of dextran 70 ranged from 600 ml to 800 ml. The main differences between these two solutions concern their influence on microcirculation. Infusion of dextran 40 has been described to increase microcirculatory flow because of a reduced red cell and platelet sludging, volume expansion, and hemodilution-induced reduction in whole blood viscosity. Dextrans are associated with anaphylactic reactions, coagulation abnormalities, and impaired blood cross-matching [8].

Gelatin exists in different modifications, e.g., modified fluid gelatin and ureabridged gelatin. The only major differences between these preparations consist in different electrolyte concentrations. The increase of blood volume is approximately the same as that of the infused volume of gelatin (range 70% to 90%). Due to the low MW (LMW) average (approximately 35,000), plasma half-life is rather short (2–3 h) and reinfusion is necessary to maintain adequate blood volume. Thus, with regard to volume effect, gelatins are the least effective colloid. The definite incidence of (severe) anaphylactic reaction mediated by gelatin induced histamin liberation is still not completely known [14].

Various types of HES preparations with different concentrations (3%, 6%, 10%), different weight averages (MW) (70,000, 200,000, 450,000 dalton) and different degrees of molar substitution ratio (MS) (0.5, 0.62, 0.7) are used. Moreover, there is convincing evidence that the activity of the alpha-amylase depends on the position of the hydroxyethyl groups on the glucose molecule (C_2, C_3, C_6). The ratio of the C_2:C_6 hydroxyethylation appears to be a key factor concerning the pharmcokinetic behavior of HES and possibly also for its side effects. Unfortunately, today the C_2:C_6 ratio is not shown by the manufacturers. The extent and duration of plasma expansion are extremely dependent on the physical and chemical characteristics of the HES solution [15]. Comparison of the different studies using HES solutions is difficult, because they vary widely concerning the subjects studied, rate and amount of infused volume, and endpoint of fluid therapy. The answer to the question as to which is the best HES solution to optimize macro- and microcirculation in the criticilly ill warrants further investigations.

Fluid Therapy and Regulators of Perfusion

Composition and volume of each body compartment are controlled through a complex mechanism which includes the antidiuretic system (ADH), renin-aldosterone-angiotensin (RAA), and the sympathetic nervous system. The principal actions of these systems are to retain water in order to restore water or intravascular volume deficit, to retain sodium in order to restore the intravascular volume, and to increase the hydrostatic perfusion pressure through vasoconstriction. The control of ADH secretion depends on plasmatic osmolality, whereas the most important stimulus for activation of the RAA system is depletion of the intravascular volume. However, enhanced activity of ADH, RAA, and catecholamines is known to occur in stress situations, e.g., during surgery. Although the normal response to surgery and starvation results in improved metabolic activity, it can be expected that a pre-existing deficit of water or intravascular volume further increases this activity. If the stimulus of water or intravascular volume deficit and the stress-related stimulus of ADH, RAA, and catecholamines is additive, fluid management could inhibit them through a counter-regulatory mechanism. Several attempts to inhibit or attenuate the activity of ADH and RAA systems by administering different volumes of isotonic crystalloid solutions were made. However, it is known that the ADH production is subordinated to the maintenance of the extracellular volume and, in particular, the intravascular compartment. Administration of a restricted volume of crystalloid solutions could possibly replace a previous deficit of water, but the replacement of a previous deficit of intravascular volume would require much more volume in order to inhibit the secretory stimulus of all the regulators committed to maintain it. Thus the replacement of water alone will not inhibit the normal response of ADH and RAA, whereas administration of a combination of crystalloid and colloid solutions (replacement of water deficit simultaneously with improvement of the effective intravascular volume) may achieve this goal.

Restoration of flow is an essential key for avoiding tissue ischemia and subsequent development of multiple organ failure (MOF) [16]. A point of controversy in this area appears to be the question as to which kind of solution is best suitable to avoid the sequelae of trauma or surgery. The effects of long-term infusion (over 5 days) of exclusively either albumin 20% or 10% HES 200/0.5 on important regulators of macro- and microcirculation were studied in trauma and septic surgical patients [17]. In trauma patients, concentrations of important vasoactive substances showed an almost similar course in both groups. In both sepsis groups, however, plasma levels of vasopressors (vasopressin, endothelin-1, norepinephrine, and epinephrine) were significantly elevated beyond normal. Within the investigation period they decreased more pronouncedly in the HES- than in the albumin-treated patients. Atrial natriuretic peptide (ANP) increased in the albumin patients, 6-keto-prostaglandin F 1alpha plasma levels (the stable but inactive end product of prostaglandin I 2 [prostacyclin]) decreased significantly only in the HES-treated sepsis patients. Summarizing the results, it can be assumed that volume replacement with albumin 20% and 10% HES 200/0.5 in trauma patients resulted in similar plasma levels of important regulators of macro- and microcirculation. In sepsis patients, plasma levels of these regulators were more beneficially modified by volume replacement with HES than by albumin infusion. Although macrocirculation did not differ significantly in this study, it may result in beneficial effects on tissue organ perfusion.

Volume Therapy in Particular Situations

Cardiac Surgery Patients

Absolute or relative blood volume deficits often occur during cardiac surgery. Bleeding may cause absolute volume deficit vasodilation mediated by vasodilating substances (e.g., nitroglycerin, protamin) are involved in producing relative volume deficit. Moreover, within the first 24 h after cardiac operations, a reduction in blood and plasma volume is a common phenomenon [18].

In patients undergoing major, long-lasting procedures using cardiopulmonary bypass (CPB) stable hemodynamics appear to be a prerequisite to avoid postoperative organ dysfunction. When discussing different ways of volume therapy in cardiac patients, not only macrocirculatory effects have to be taken into account, but influence on pulmonary function, rheological abnormalities, and alteration of coagulation are also of equal importance. Progressive respiratory insufficiency after operations using CPB has been termed "post-perfusion lung syndrome." It is characterized by an increasing fluid accumulation in the pulmonary tissue with consecutive deterioration of the pulmonary gas exchange. One of the fundamental lesions in this disease is an abnormal increase in pulmonary endothelial permeability. This alteration in capillary integrity may be related to the effects of pump oxygenators and synthetic nonendothelial surfaces on blood components. The release of various kinins and other vasoactive substances may also be due to the unphysiologic perfusion during CPB. Perioperative myocardial ischemia may also influence endothelial permeability. Last but not least, depressed left ventricular performance after CPB will synergistically influence fluid flux across a damaged pulmonary microvascular membrane. Imbalance between extravasation of fluid from the pulmonary microcirculation and the ability of pulmonary lymphatics to remove excess fluid result in lung water accumulation. Both myocardial performance and susceptibility of the endothelial integrity are changed in the elderly and critically ill patient, so that the choice of fluid therapy has to be considered carefully. Crystalloids alone seem to be less qualified for volume replacement because of the large amount which is necessary to guarantee hemodynamic stability. Stein et al. [19] demonstrated that 70% of elderly patients suffering from circulatory shock and having received crystalloids for volume stabilization developed pulmonary edema, in contrast to 25% of a colloid-treated group. Thus, there seems to be an increased risk to older patients of deterioration of pulmonary function by infusion of crystalloids in this situation.

With regard to Starling's equation, colloid oncotic pressure (COP) seems to play a major role in the maintenance of pulmonary fluid balance. Several authors could demonstrate that a decrease in COP was followed by a compromised pulmonary function in critically ill patients, and they concluded that application of albumin might reduce these complications [20–22]. The administration of large volumes of albumin, however, has been associated with detrimental effects on pulmonary function. Virgilio et al. [23] reported on deteriorated pulmonary gas exchange after albumin administration in patients suffering from shock. In the case of impaired integrity of the pulmonary capillary membrane, albumin may leak rapidly into the interstitial space and can have an "inverse" deleterious oncotic effect. In a study in cardiac surgery patients, it was demonstrated that albumin administration after CPB was followed by a deteriorated pulmonary function because of an increase in extravascular lung water (EVLW) [24].

Fluid Therapy in Children

Although synthetic colloids have replaced albumin in several centers as the first choice for volume replacement in the adult critically ill, albumin remains the most widely used fluid for volume therapy in children. Only very limited studies on the use of synthetic colloids in children are available. In a study in children undergoing pediatric cardiac surgery, 6% HES 200,000/0.5 has been compared with albumin [25]. Hemodynamics were sufficiently restored with both fluids, and coagulation parameters and laboratory values were without differences among these two groups. It was concluded that LMW-HES solution can effectively and safely be used for volume replacement, even in small children undergoing cardiac surgery.

Side Effects of Volume Replacement

Theoretical and documented hazards are associated with each kind of volume therapy. This cannot explain the emotional atmosphere of the discussion about the "ideal" solution for volume replacement.

There is concern that some synthetic colloids may have an adverse effect on hemostasis. The mechanisms by which synthetic colloids may exert platelet-inhibiting effects have not been fully elucidated. When using dextran, both VIIIR:Ag and VIIIR:RCo levels decrease significantly. With reduced VIIIR:RCo, there is reduced binding to the platelet membrane receptor proteins GPIb and GPIIb/IIIa, which results in a decreased platelet adhesion. The effects of the various preparations of HES have so far been only partially defined. Both normal and abnormal platelet aggregation were reported. HMW-HES (450/0.7) diminished the concentrations of VIIIR:Ag and VIIIR:RCo more pronouncedly than HES with LMW-HES. In a study in cardiac surgery patients, it was shown that HMW-HES resulted overall in the most pronounced impairment of platelet aggregation and should be avoided in patients with an increased risk of higher postoperative bleeding [26]. LMW-HES did not show the same negative effects on platelet aggregation as were seen in the HMW-HES group. It is of particular importance that albumin, which is favored in many centers, was not different from LMW-HES with regard to platelet function, post-bypass bleeding, and the need for allogeneic blood.

The metabolism of the fluids used for volume therapy is not definitely known. Gelatin is rapidly eliminated by the kidneys (MW 35,000). Direct assay of gelatin or possible metabolites is difficult, and thus it is not definitely clear what happens with this colloid. Dextrans are not metabolized intravascularly. The kidney filters smaller molecular fractions; larger fractions pass to tissues and undergo complete hydrolysis by dextran-1,6 glucosidase. HES undergoes a slow intravascular catabolism by a-amylase. The smaller molecules are rapidly eliminated by glomerular filtration. Depending on the kind of HES solution (especially on the MS and on the C_2/C_6 ratio), a varying degree of the infused HES leaves the vascular department and is taken up by the reticuloendothelial system (=accumulation of starch). Apparently this does not affect its function [27]. Final elimination is very slow, and the long-term effect of this persistance is not clearly known.

Monitoring of Fluid Therapy in the Critically Ill

Points of controversy in this area appear on the question of which monitoring measure is the best to guide volume therapy. It is imperative that critically ill surgical patients receiving volume therapy are adequately monitored to avoid and detect signs of "fluid failure" early. Low arterial blood pressure partly associated with an increased heart rate is the most obvious sign of low output. The hypovolemic patient additionally may have a low central venous pressure (CVP) and pulmonary capillary wedge pressure (PCWP). However, hemodynamic data vary widely and are markedly dependent on the underlying disease and concomitant medication (e.g., beta-blockers). Patients with altered ventricular compliance may have high CVP although volume deficit exists. The initial approach is to challenge the patient with a volume load. Pump failure is present when a sufficient preload has been achieved and blood flow is still not adequately distributed to meet the tissues' metabolic requirements.

The problem of which is the best method to monitor "load" is still unsolved. Particularly in patients with altered ventricular compliance, commonly monitored parameters such CVP, right atrial pressure (RAP), or right ventricular pressure (RVP) not always proved valid enough to judge loading conditions, thus supporting the premise that the preload factor in the original Frank-Starling hypothesis has nothing to do with pressure.

The perioperatively cardiovascular unstable patient is at risk of experiencing significant splanchnic hypoperfusion with subsequent development of translocation and eventually multiple organ failure (MOF) [28, 29]. Gastric intramucosal pH (pHi) measurement has emerged as an attractive option for diagnosis and monitoring of splanchnic hypoperfusion. In patients undergoing major noncardiac surgery, maintaining hemodynamic stability was no guarantee of adequate splanchnic perfusion and could not definitely protect against significant postoperative complications [30]. Monitoring of pHi had greater importance for predicting postoperative complications (sensitivity 93.3%, specifity 50%). Although this monitoring instrument has produced some promising results, it is far from being the new "gold standard" for guiding patients' management, including volume administration.

Conclusion

Adequate volume therapy is known to be a therapeutic cornerstone in the critically ill. A substantial body of evidence supports the concept that deterioration in systemic and regional perfusion (e.g., splanchnic perfusion) may be of particular importance for development of perioperative complications. Thus, volume replacement should not only be focused on restoration of macrocirculation, but microcirculation should be improved as well.

The choice of fluid for volume replacement is influenced by various factors. Perfusion, organ function, and endothelial integrity can be restored more rapidly with colloid than with crystalloid solutions. Massive crystalloid resuscitation alone is less likely to achieve adequate restoration of blood flow and tissue O_2. When comparing albumin and synthetic colloids, several studies have demonstrated no differences between these colloids. The major advantage of synthetic colloids is in their relative economy. Although cost considerations are very difficult because of different medical systems in different countries, treatment with albumin is markedly more expensive than fluid therapy with synthetic colloids, and routine use of albumin for volume therapy cannot be justified in the surgical or intensive care patient.

Several studies have revisited the crystalloid–colloid controversy [31–33] – results, however, are still conflicting. It has been questioned whether meta-analyses are helpful to examine the effects of crystalloid or colloid fluid resuscitation on mortality [34], because mortality was never the endpoint of any of the crystalloid/colloid studies. Mortality does not seem to be an appropriate endpoint when comparing these two volume replacement regimens. Endpoints need to focus on organ function, inflammation, or perfusion rather than on outcome.

References

1. Shoemaker WC, Appel PL, Kram HB, Waxman K, Lee TS (1988) Prospective trial of supranormal values of survivors as therapeutic goals in high-risk surgical patients. Chest 94:1176–1186
2. Boyd O, Grounds RM, Bennet ED (1993) A randomized clinical trial of the effect of deliberate perioperative increase of oxygen delivery on mortality in high-risk surgical patients. JAMA 270:2699–2707
3. Prough DS, Johnston WE (1989) Fluid restoration in septic shock: no solution yet. Anesth Analg 69:699–704
4. Davidson I (1989) Fluid resuscitation of shock: current controversies. Crit Care Med 17:1078–1080
5. Haljamäe H (1993) Volume substitution in shock. Acta Anaesthesiol Scand 37 [Suppl 98]:25–28
6. Stockwell MA, Scott A, Day A, Riley B, Soni N (1992) Colloid solutions in the critically ill. Anaesthesia 47:3–9
7. Beards SC, Watt T, Edwards JD, Nightingale P, Farragher EB (1994) Comparison of the hemodynamic and oxygen transport responses to modified fluid gelatin and hetastarch in critically ill patients: a prospective, randomized trial. Crit Care Med 22:600–605
8. Kreimeier U, Peter K (1998) Strategies of volume therapy in sepsis and systemic inflammatory response syndrome. Kidney Int 53 [Suppl 64]:75–79
9. Zornow MH, Prough DS (1995) Fluid management in patients with traumatic brain injury. New Horizons 3:488–498
10. Edwards JD (1994) A new debate: colloid versus colloid? In: Vincent JL (ed) Yearbook of intensive care and emergency medicine. Springer, Berlin Heidelberg New York, pp 152–164
11. Lamke LO, Liljedahl SO (1976) Plasma volume changes after infusion of various plasma expanders. Resuscitation 5:93–98
12. Vaupshas HJ, Levy M (1990) Distribution of saline following acute volume loading: postural effects. Clin Invest Med 13:165
13. Neumann M, Demling RH (1990) Colloid vs crystalloid: a current perspective. Intensive Crit Care Dig 9:3–5
14. Laxenaire M, Charpentier C, Feldman L (1994) Reactions anaphylactoides aux subitutes colloidaux du plasma: incidence, facteurs de risque, mecanismes. Ann Fr Anest Reanimat 13:301–310
15. Quon CF (1988) Clinical pharmacokinetics and pharmacodynamics of colloidal plasma volume expanders. J Cardiothorac Anesth 2 [Suppl 1]:13–23

16. Sibbald WJ (1994) Fluid therapy in sepsis. In: Reinhard K, Eyrich K, Sprung C (eds) Sepsis – current perspectives in pathophysiology and therapy. Springer, Berlin Heidelberg New York, pp 266–273 (Update in Intensive care and emergency medicine, vol 18)
17. Boldt J, Müller M, Mentges D, Papsdorf M, Hempelmann G (1996) Influence of different volume therapy regime on regulators of circulation in the critically ill. Br J Anaesth 77:480–487
18. Karanko MS, Klossner JA, Laaksonen VO (1987) Restoration of volume by crystalloids versus colloid after coronary artery bypass: hemodynamics, lung water, oxygenation, and outcome. Crit Care Med 15:559–566
19. Stein L, Berand J, Morisette M (1975) Pulmonary edema during volume infusion. Circulation 52:483–489
20. Rackow EC, Fein A, Leppo J (1977) Colloid osmotic pressure as a prognostic indicator of pulmonary edema and mortality in the critical ill. Chest 72:709–713
21. Weil MH, Henning RJ, Puroi VK (1979) Colloid oncotic pressure: clinical significance. Crit Care Med 7:113–120
22. Morissette M, Weil HW, Shubin H (1975) Reduction in colloid osmotic pressure associated with fatal progression of cardiopulmonary failure. Crit Care Med 3:115–120
23. Virgilio RW, Rice C, Smith D (1979) Crystalloid vs colloid resuscitation: Is one better? Surg 2:129–135
24. Boldt J, v Bormann B, Kling D, Börner U, Mulch J, Hempelmann G (1985) Colloidosmotic pressure and extravascular lung water after extracorporeal circulation. Herz 10:366–375
25. Boldt J, Knothe Ch, Schindler E, Hammermann H, Dapper F, Hempelmann G (1993): Volume replacement with hydroxyethyl starch solution in children. Br J Anaesth 70:661–665
26. Boldt J, Knothe Ch, Zickmann B, Andres P, Dapper F, Hempelmann G (1993) Influence of different intravascular volume therapy on platelet function in patients undergoing cardiopulmonary bypass. Anesth Analg 76:1185–1190
27. Lackner FX, Graninger W, Illias W, Panzer S, Schulz E (1990) Präoperative Eigenblutspende, der Einfluß von Hydroxyäthylstärke auf Rekuloendothelialsystem und Opsonine. Infusionstherapie 17:276
28. Fiddian-Green RG (1990) Gut mucosal ischaemia during cardiac surgery. In: Taylor K (ed) Seminars in cardiovascular surgery. Saunders, Philadelphia, pp 1–11
29. Mythen MG, Webb AR (1994) The role of gut mucosal hypoperfusion in the pathogenesis of postoperative organ dysfunction. Intensive Care Med 20:203–209
30. Mythen MG, Webb AR (1995) Perioperative plasma volume expansion reduces the incidence of gut mucosal hypoperfusion during cardiac surgery. Ann Surg 130:423–429
31. Velanovich V (1989) Crystalloid versus colloid fluid resuscitation: a meta-analysis of mortality. Surgery 105:65–71
32. Schlierhout G, Roberts I (1998) Fluid resuscitation with colloids or crystalloids in critically ill patients: a systematic review of randomised trials. BMJ 316:961–964
33. Cochrane injuries group albumin reviewers (1998) Human albumin administration in critically ill patients: systematic review of randomised controlled trials. BMJ 317:235–239
34. Astiz ME, Rackow EC (1999) Crystalloid-colloid controversy revisited. Crit Care Med 27:34–35

CHAPTER 7

Efficacy of Plasma Substitutes for Volume Therapy

J. TREIB, M.T. GRAUER, A. HAASS

Introduction

Plasma substitutes are used in the prophylaxis and treatment of hypovolemia due the loss of blood and plasma after surgery, trauma, burns or infections (London et al. 1989, Shoemaker and Kram 1990, Baron and Treib 1998). Another area of use is hemodilution therapy, carried out in cerebral, retinal, otogenic and peripheral perfusion disorders (Kiesewetter et al. 1987, Haaß et al. 1991, Remky et al. 1994, Hansen et al. 1995). Placenta insufficiency and coronary heart disease are additional possible indications (Koscielny et al. 1991, Molendijk et al. 1995, Bsteh et al. 1995).

Crystalloid solutions are the most frequently used plasma substitutes (Shoemaker and Kram 1990). They are cheap and can be used without the danger of anaphylactic reactions. Crystalloids are used for the treatment of dehydration, increase urinary output and interstitial fluid. Albumin, Fresh Frozen Plasma (FFP), Plasma Protein Fraction (PPF) and non-protein colloids such as hydroxyethyl starch (HES), Dextran and Gelatin are used alternatively instead of a high-dose infusion of crystalloids. This is particularly the case if the main goal is the increase of intravascular volume, for example in the therapy of acute blood loss or during hemodilution. Compared to crystalloids, colloids cause only a small increase of interstitial fluid and result therefore in a smaller post-ischemic brain edema (Shoemaker and Kram 1990, Matsui et al. 1993).

For hemodilution therapy, mostly colloidal plasma substitutes are used, because the infusion of crystalloids alone does not lower hematocrit effectively nor increase cardiac output (CO) (Appel et al. 1981, Hankeln et al. 1989). Staedt (1994) was able to show in patients with acute ischemic stroke that hematocrit remained constant after an infusion of 500 ml of Ringer solution, whereas an infusion of 500 ml 10% HES 200/0.5 lowered hematocrit significantly. The hemodynamic parameters heart frequency, blood pressure, stroke volume and CO also remained constant after infusion of Ringer solution, while the infusion of a starch solution increased significantly blood pressure (+6%), stroke volume (+11%) and CO (+14%).

This explains why Funk and Baldinger (1995) observed in animal microscopic invivo studies that microcirculatory perfusion remained stable during an isovolemic hemodilution with Dextran 60, whereas tissue perfusion and oxygenation was impaired after bloodletting and high-dose infusion of Ringer solution.

For cardiac operations, burns, sepsis and larger surgery, artificial colloids such as HES, Dextran and Gelatin were shown to be as safe and efficacious as albumin solutions (Rackow et al. 1989, Camu et al. 1995). Several groups observed a larger increase in CO after infusion of 10% medium molecular weight HES than after infusion of 5% albumin solution, which can be attributed to a greater plasma-expanding effect of starch solution (London et al. 1989, Waxman et al. 1989, Hankeln et al. 1990). Therefore, the use of albumin as a plasma expander alone is not advisable anymore. Because of occasionally occurring albumin shortages and for reasons of cost-effectiveness and infectious risk, which cannot be excluded with certainty, artificial colloids (such as low-molecular weight or medium molecular weight starches or Gelatin) are a better choice in volume therapy than albumin, as long as protein concentration in the blood is above 3–4 g/dl (Hankeln et al. 1990). The indications for the use of albumin should be reconsidered under new aspects, such as substance-specific effects of albumin itself that go beyond the osmotic effects. Very little data is available about this and more studies need to be conducted in the future to establish these albumin-specific indications.

Regarding their effects on hemodynamics and oxygen transport, the different artificial colloids are very similar, as long as the volume effect is comparable (Beards et al. 1994, Staedt 1994). Because of the great therapeutic safety after a one-time infusion of 500 ml to 1000 ml, HES, Gelatin and Dextran are the most frequently used artificial colloidal volume substitutes. HES and Dextran differ in their chemical structure, metabolization and elimination. This is of decisive importance for their biological effects, because the actual in-vivo effect of a plasma substitute is determined by the composition and nature of the molecules that are generated through the in-vivo metabolism.

HES is a high-polymer glucose compound. It is manufactured through hydrolysis and subsequent hydroxyethylation of the highly-branched starch amylopectin. HES consists of glucose units that are linked within the chain through alpha-1,4 and at the branching points through alpha-1,6 glycosidic bonds (Fig. 1).

Initially, starch solutions were characterized only through their initial molecular weight, i.e. through their weight averaged molecular weight (Mw), measured in-vitro. However, the determination of the initial molecular weight alone is not sufficient, because HES is broken down in-vivo.

The molar substitution ratio describes the average number of hydroxyethyl groups per glucose unit. 10% HES 200/0.62 has a concentration of 10%, a medium initial molecular weight of 200,000 D and 62% of its glucose units have a hydroxyethyl group attached to them. The alpha-amylases in the blood can only break down unsubstituted glucose units. Changing the degree of substitution allows control over the rate of enzymatic breakdown and with it control over the extent and duration of the volume effect.

Because substitution is possible at the carbon 2, 3 or 6 of the glucose molecule, different substitution patterns exist. The substitution pattern can be characterized through the C2/C6 hydroxyethylation ratio. The higher this ratio, i.e. the higher the share of glucose molecules that are substituted at the C2 atom, the slower the starch is metabolized (Yoshida et al. 1973 and 1984), leading to a different in-vivo effect of the starch (Treib et al. 1995 and 1996).

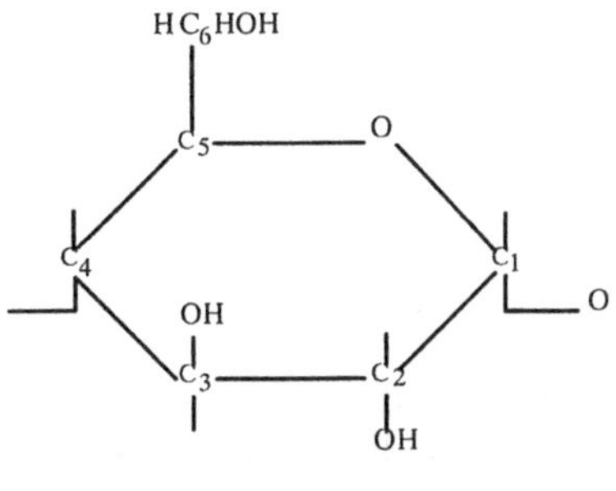

Fig. 1. Anhydroglucose unit with alpha-1,4 glycosidic bond

Table 1. Characterization of commonly used Dextran and hydroxyethylstarch solutions

Dextran	
Concentration	6%; 10%
Initial molecular weight	40000; 60000; 70000; 75000
Hydroxyethyl starch (HES)	
Concentration	6%; 10%
Initial molecular weight	70000; 130000; 200000; 450000
degree of substitution	0.4; 0.5; 0.62; 0.7
C2/C6-ration	4–13

Dextrans are long-chain macromolecules with little branching that are hardly metabolized. Their elimination is mostly renal, with the elimination rate depending on the size of the molecules (Kroemer et al. 1987).

Dextrans are available in concentrations of 6% and 10%. The mean Mw can be 40,000 D; 60,000 D or 75,000 D. Starches are available as 6% and 10% solutions, whose mean initial molecular weight can be 70,000, 200,000 or 450,000 D. In addition, degree of substitution and the pattern of substitution can vary (Table 1).

Initially, hemodilution therapy was mostly carried with low molecular weight Dextrans, because they were thought to have favorable rheological properties (Gottstein 1969). After Haaß et al. (1996) and Kroemer et al. (1987) were able to show that Dextran 40 loses its favorable rheological properties after repeated administration because of the accumulation of macromolecules, starch solutions gained popularity.

Because of their long-lasting volume effect, high molecular weight starch solutions, such as Hetastarch with a Mw of 450,000 D, were more popular in the beginning, particularly in the United States. However, after repeated infusion or the infusion of larger volumes, hemorrhagic complications were observed in individual cases (Symington 1986, Damon et al. 1987, Bianchine 1987, Cully et al. 1987, Abramson 1988, Lockwood et al. 1988). Recently, Trumble et al. (1995) reported the increased occurrence of hemorrhagic complications after infusion of Hetastarch during vasospasm treatment in patients with subarachnoid hemorrhage. Because of this, Trumble et al. advised against infusions of HES and recommended instead the use of Plasma Protein Fraction (PPF).

Hemostasiological studies showed that the hemorrhages observed under Hetastarch were caused by an acquired von Willebrand syndrome (Stump et al. 1985, Sanfelippo et al. 1988). Strauss and colleagues (1988) obsered that medium molecular weight starch (Pentastarch, Mw 264 kD) has fewer unfavorable effects on coagulation than high molecular weight starch. In addition, medium molecular weight starch has better rheological properties and remains for a shorter time in the human body (Mishler 1980, Köhler et al. 1982, Haaß et al. 1986 and 1992, Kroemer et al. 1987). This increased the popularity of medium molecular weight starches in Europe.

The effects of a one-time administration of the different colloidal plasma substitutes on rheology and coagulation have been studied repeatedly (Karlson et al. 1967, Landgraf et al. 1981, Ehrly et al. 1985, Kiesewetter et al. 1986, Scheffler et al. 1987, Jung et al. 1988 and 1989). The effects of a repeated infusion of larger volumes, such as during a hemodynamically oriented volume therapy, have not been studied sufficiently, although more pronounced effects are to be expected. A long-term volume therapy is a good model to judge therapeutic safety of plasma substitutes, because possible side effects will show more clearly due to the much higher doses.

Particularly in the volume therapy of cerebral circulation disorders it is important to use a plasma substitute which affects coagulation as little as possible. Initiation of therapy can proceed much more rapidly, because an intracerebral hemorrhage does not have to be excluded by cranial CT, which has been demanded by Hartmann (1987) before initiating a treatment with Dextran 40.

Patients and Methods

After obtaining informed consent, we carried out a hypervolemic hemodilution therapy in 74 patients with cerebral perfusion disorders (Haaß et al. 1991, Treib et al. 1995–1997). No patient suffered from a manifest cardiac or renal insufficiency.

Infusion Solutions

Infused plasma substitutes included 10% Dextran 40 (NaCl-free), 6% and 10% HES 200/0.62 (C2/C6 ratio = 9) and 6% HES 70/0.5 (C2/C6 ratio = 4). In addition, we infused three derivates of a 10% HES 200/0.5 solution with different C2/C6 ratios: HES 200/05 (C2/C6 ratio = 5) and two HES solutions that were identical except for their pattern of substitution (both manufactured by the same manufacturer), in the following called 10% HES 200/0.5 (1) and (2). The C2/C6 ratio for 10% HES 200/0.5 (1) was 13.4 and for HES 200/0.5 (2) it was 5.7.

Infusion Protocols

All patients received initially a rapid infusion of a "loading dose" 500 ml plasma expander and 500 ml electrolyte solution. The subsequent protocol showed only minor differences for the individual substances. For HES 200/0.62 a smaller total dose was chosen, because this starch has a longer-lasting volume effect due to its higher degree of substitution (Table 2).

Methods of Measurement

Hematocrit was measured with a hematocrit centrifuge. A measuring capillary containing heparin was filled with blood and closed at the bottom. After centrifugation for 5 minutes, hematocrit was determined with a normogramm from the quotient: height of the cellular column divided by the total height of the column.

Erythrocyte aggregation was determined with the hematocrit erythrocyte desaggregation device HEDA (manufactured by Rheomed GmbH, Germany) (Kiesewetter et al. 1982). Erythrocyte aggregates were dispersed at sedimentation degrees of over 500/s. After stopping dispersion, the reproducible decline in the optical

Table 2. Infusion protocols (Haaß et al. 1991, Treib et al. 1995–1997)

10% HES 200/0.5	
Day 1–4:	1000 ml HES over 24 hours with 1000 ml electrolyte solution
Day 5–10:	500 ml HES over 12 hours with 500 ml electrolyte solution
10% Dextran 40	
Day 1–4:	1000 ml Dextran over 12 hours with 1000 ml electrolyte solution
Day 5–10:	500 ml Dextran with 500 ml electrolyte solution
10% HES 200/0.62:	
Day 1–9/10:	500 ml HES over 12 hours with 500 ml electrolyte solution
6% HES 200/0.62	
Day 1–4:	1000 ml HES over 24 hours
Day 5–9/10:	500 ml HES over 12 hours
6% HES 70/0.5:	
Day 1–4:	1000 ml HES over 24 hours with 1000 ml electrolyte solution
Day 5–10:	500 ml HES over 12 hours with 500 ml electrolyte solution

density of the standing blood is the result of renewed aggregation of erythrocytes. The tendency of the erythrocytes to aggregate was computed from the time curve describing the decline in optical density.

To measure plasma viscosity, a capillary tube plasma viscosimeter was used (KSPV 3, manufactured by Rheomed GmbH, Germany) (Jung et al. 1983). A plasma bolus situated in a standardized capillary tube at 37°C was set in motion by cutting the tube at the upper end. Photo diodes measured the time needed for the plasma bolus to move over a defined length. Using calibrated scales, plasma viscosity was computed using the time of passage.

HES serum concentration was measured with the hexokinase and o-toluidine method (Förster et al. 1981). Serum was mixed with concentrated base and boiled. Grain alcohol was added and the mixture shaken. After cooling and centrifugation, the supernatant was removed. The precipitate was taken up with hydrochloric acid and incubated in boiling water. After another cooling step, glucose was measured in the hydrolysate with hexokinase-glucose-6-phosphate dehydrogenase and o-toluidine.

HES molecular weight distribution was measured using exclusion chromatography, combined with small-angle laser light diffraction (Eigner 1988). The mean molecular weight (Mw), the molecular weight of the 10% largest and smallest molecules, the average of the molar mass (Mn) and the width of molecular weight distribution were determined (Mw/Mn).

Platelet number and volume was determined with the Whole-Blood-Platelet-Analyzer 810 (manufactured by Baker Instruments) and Sysmex M-2000 (manufactured by Digitana AG) with electric resistance measurements. Platelet aggregation was measured with an Eppendorf photometer PAT III-1101 M (Bredding et al. 1975). A rotation-induced spontaneous aggregation of platelets can be measured photometrically, because beginning platelet aggregation in platelet-rich plasma can observed through an increase in light transparency. This event was registered with a photometer and recorded. Rotation time of the disc-cuvette was 15 minutes. Measure for the maximum aggregation velocity was angle alpha-2 between the tanget at the maximum decline of the aggregation curve and the horizontal.

Thromboplastin time (quick) was measured after the method by Biggs and MacFarlain (1962). The quick test examines the activity of the extrinsic system and factors II, V, VII, X. The calcium-thromboplastin reagent by Boeringer Mannheim GmbH and a coagulometer manufactured by Amelung GmbH was used. After adding tissue thromboplastin and calcium, prothrombin becomes thrombin via the extrinsic system of the plasma. The time until the occurrence of coagulation was determined with the coagulometer. The result was recorded in per cent relation to normal plasma scale. Reference range (industry standard) was 70%–120%.

Partial thromboplastin time (PTT) was measured according to the method by Larrieu and Weiland (1957). The coagulometer KC 10 and the aPTT reagent by Boeringer Mannheim GmbH (Böttcher et al. 1979) was used. The PTT test serves to examine the intrinsic system of the coagulation and factors VIII, IX, XI, XII. After addition of partial thromboplastins, surface-active substances and calcium to the plasma, thrombin is generated via the intrinsic system, which turns fibrinogen into fibrin. The reference range according to industry standards was 26–40 seconds.

Thrombin time was measured with the coagulometer KC 10 and reagents by Boeringer Mannheim GmbH, using the method by Biggs and MacFarlain (1962). After adding the enzyme thrombin to the plasma, fibrinogen becomes fibrin. The thrombin time is the directly measured coagulation time. Reference range according to industry standards was 16–20 seconds.

Fibrinogen concentration was measured using fibrinogen reagents from Boeringer Mannheim GmbH and the coagulometer KC 10 after the method by Clauss (1957). Citrate plasma was strongly diluted to minimize the influence of factors that affect coagulation. To the diluted citrate plasma thrombin was added, and the time until the occurrence of a fibrin clot measured. Industry standard reference range was 150–450 mg/dl.

Factors II, V, VII, VIII:C, IX, X, XI and XII were measured with the coagulometer KC 10 and corresponding plasma reagents from Immuno GmbH (Heidelberg, Germany). Citrate plasma was strongly diluted to minimize the influence of factors affecting coagulation. To the citrate plasma, the corresponding plasma was added, which contained an excess of all coagulation factors except the one to be tested for. The time until the occurrence of coagulation depends on the activity of the studied coagulation factor. According to industry standards, the following reference ranges were used: factor II: 70–130%, factor V: 70–140%, Factor VIII:C: 70–200%, factor IX: 70–110%, factor X: 70–140%, factor XI: 80–120% and factor XII: 80–120%.

Von Willebrand Ristocetin co-factor was measured using the protocol and reagents of the Behringwerke AG, Marburg, Germany. Stabilized platelets were agglutinated in the presence of von Willebrand Ristocetin co-factor and the antibiotic ristocetin, to examine the function of the factor. Industry standard reference range was 50–150%.

Von Willebrand Factor antigen, also called factor VIII-associated antigen was measured with an ELISA by Boeringer Mannheim GmbH. For the photometric measurements the Mini-Reader, manufactured by Dynatech was used. Concentrations of the von Willebrand Factor antigen were measured with an enzyme immuno assay (sandwich principle, Schlegelberger et al. 1984). During the first incubation step, a specific antibody was bound on a plastic plate. This antibody binds in a first immune reaction to the von Willebrand Factor of the sample, which has several antigenic determinants. In a second immune reaction, von Willebrand Factor antibodies marked with peroxidase form sandwich complexes, which are a measure for the activity of the factor. In the following washing step, un-bound peroxidase conjugate is removed. Activity of bound peroxidase is measured photometrically. Industry standard reference range is 60–150%.

Multimeric analysis of the von Willebrand factor was carried out with sodium dodecyl sulfate (SDS) agarose gel electrophoresis (Ruggeri and Zimmermann 1981, Budde und Steinberg 1985). The plasma samples were diluted 1:5 with SDS-containing sample buffer and incubated for 30 minutes at 60°C. Of each sample solution, 25 µl were plated on the agarose gel plate (Sigma, Deisenhofen and Biozyn, Hameln, Germany). Disc electrophoresis was carried out for one hour at 16°C with 25 mA/gel and for 15 hours with 15 mA/gel. After western blotting, the samples were incubated with rabbit-anti-human von Willebrand factor (A-082 Dakopatts, Hamburg, Germany). After repeated washing, swine anti-rabbit immunoglobulin (Z-196 Dakopatts, Hamburg, Germany) was used as second antibody. The third antibody was peroxidase-conjugated plasmin anti-plasmin rabbit antibody (Z-113, Dakopatts). Staining was carried out with 4-chloro-1-naphthol solution and hydrogen peroxide.

C1-inactivator concentration was measured following the protocol and using the reagents from Behringwerke AG, Marburg, Germany with simple radial immune diffusion. After a diffusion time of two days, the diameter of the precipitates was measured and compared with a reference table from the manufacturer. Reference range was from 64–146%.

C1-inactivator acitivity was measured with the protocol and the reagents from Behringwerge AG Marburg. C1-inactivator in the sample inhibits the C1 esterase that is present in excess. The remaining activity of the C1 esterase is measured in with a kinetic test (Heber et al. 1983). Reference range was from 80–125%.

Fibronectin concentration was measured with simple radial diffusion, using reagents from Behringwerke AG. After a diffusion time of two days, fibronectin concentration was determined from the diameter of the precipitate and a calibration curve. Reference range was 20–40 mg/dl.

To measure thrombin/antithrombin III complex, Enzygnost-TAT manufactured by Behringwerke AG was used. Measurements were carried out with a human-thrombin/antithrombin III enzyme immune assay (sandwich principle, Pelzer et al. 1986). Reference range was 1.0–4.1 µg/l.

Mean values and standard deviation were computed. For non-normal samples, the median was determined. To test for significance between paired samples, the Wilcoxon signed rank test was used. To test for significance between unpaired samples, the Mann-Whitney rank-sum test was used (Claus and Ebner 1985, Ramm and Hoffmann 1987).

For a more detailed discussion of patients and methods refer to the original articles (Haaß et al. 1991, Treib et al. 1995–1997).

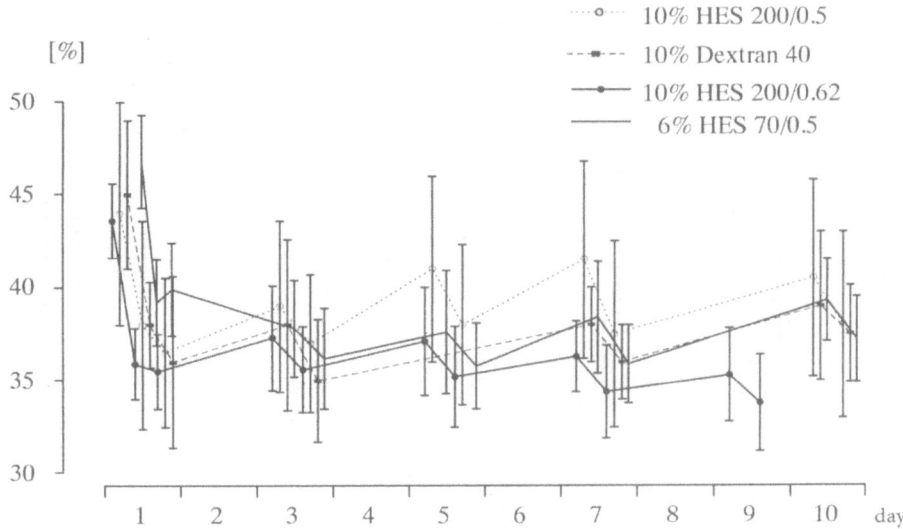

Fig. 2. Effect of a long-term infusion of 10% HES 200/0.5, 10% Dextran 40, 10% HES 200/0.62 and 6% HES 70/0.5 on hematocrit

Results

Rheological Parameters

Figure 2 shows the effect of a volume therapy with 10% HES 200/0.5, 10% Dextran 40, 10% HES 200/0.62 and 6% HES 70/0.5 on *hematocrit*. In the patient group treated with 10% HES 200/0.5, initial hematocrit was 44±5%. Until day 3, hematocrit dropped down to 36%, in the Dextran 40 group an even stronger drop from 45±3% down to 35% was observed. In the following low-dose phase, hematocrit increased slowly and on day 10, a hematocrit of 38% was measured in the group with HES 200/0.5 and 37% in the group with Dextran 40. The "loading dose" of HES 200/0.62 caused a drop in hematocrit from 43.6±2.0% to 35.9% (-17.7%). The further course of the hematocrit resembled a "see-saw" pattern. Individual infusion caused a drop in hematocrit, the following pause resulted in an increase of approximately 2 units. The lowest value was measured on day 9 at 33.8%. The dilution effect of HES 70/0.5 was smaller. For this starch, the "loading dose" led to a decrease from 46.8±2.5% to 39.2%. Through continuous infusion, this decline reached 35.5% on day 5. After reducing the amount of infusion solution by one half, hematocrit increased to 39.3%. The decrease in hematocrit was significant for all plasma substitutes (p<0.01).

The effect on the rheological parameter *erythrocyte aggregation* is displayed in Figure 3. The initial values for HES 200/0.5 and Dextran 40 were 18.3±3.5 and 21.7±3.8, respectively. For Dextran 40, erythrocyte aggregation reached 29.5 at the end of the therapy (+ 23%). This increase developed mainly during the high-dose infusion period. After dose reduction, aggregation remained stable. The individual infusions of HES 200/0.5 lowered erythrocyte aggregation more than Dextran and the tendency

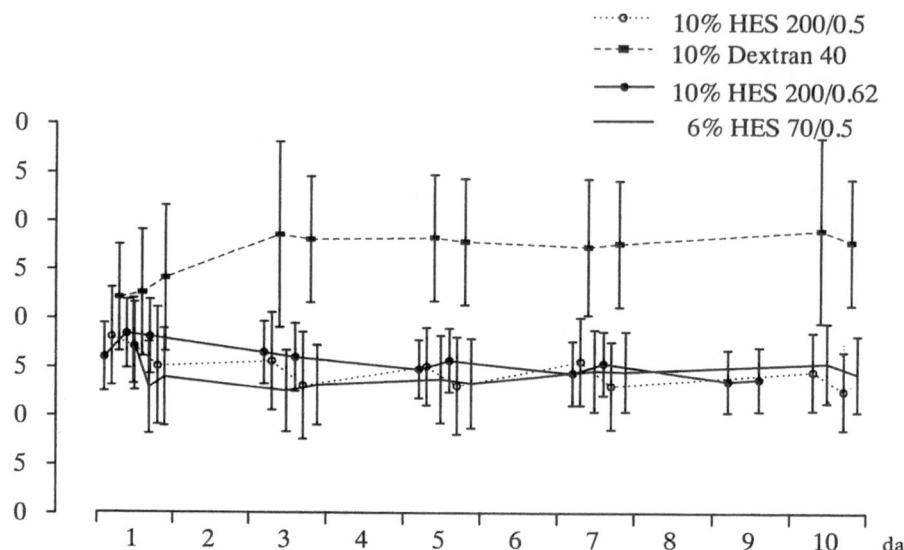

Fig. 3. Effect of a long-term infusion of 10% HES 200/0.5, 10% Dextran 40, 10% HES 200/0.62 and 6% HES 70/0.5 on erythrocyte aggregation

to aggregate was lowered continuously, reaching 14.5 on the final day, 21% below the initial value. The loading dose of the highly substituted starch (200/0.62) caused a significant (p<0.05) increase from 15.9 to 18.3 (+15.1%), which dropped continuously during the therapy, reaching the initial value on day 3, and dropping to 13.5 on the final day. The loading dose of low molecular weight HES 70/0.5 decreased the tendency to aggregate significantly (p<0.01) from 17.7 to 12.9. The lowest value was measured on day 3 at 12.6, corresponding to a decrease of 28.8%. Subsequently, the value increased again, reaching 14.4 at the end of therapy. All values were significantly (p<0.01) under the initial values.

The different plasma substitutes varied clearly in their effect on *plasma viscosity* (Fig. 4). Dextran 40 and HES 200/0.62 caused an increase during the individual infusions, which continued further. Plasma viscosity in the Dextran group was 1.38±0.06 mPas at the beginning of therapy, reaching 1.78 mPas on day 10 (+28%). HES 200/0.62 caused a continuous, significant (p<0.01) increase from 1.30±0.07 mPas to 1.54 mPas (+18.5%). Individual infusions of HES 200/0.5 and HES 70/0.5 lowered plasma viscosity. This trend continued during the therapy, the values were significantly (p<0.05) lower than the initial values of 1.36±0.05 mPas and 1.27±0.09 mPas respectively. The reduction was more long-lasting for medium molecular weight starch (5%) than for the low-molecular weight starch, which showed its maximum effect on day 3 (6%).

Measuring the *serum concentration* of the infused plasma substitutes (Fig. 5) showed an increase for Dextran 40 and the highly substituted starch during the individual infusions as well as during the whole therapy that paralleled plasma viscosity. Both substances accumulated and reached at the end of therapy a concentration of approximately 20 mg/ml. For HES 200/0.5 and HES 70/0.5 no such accumulation

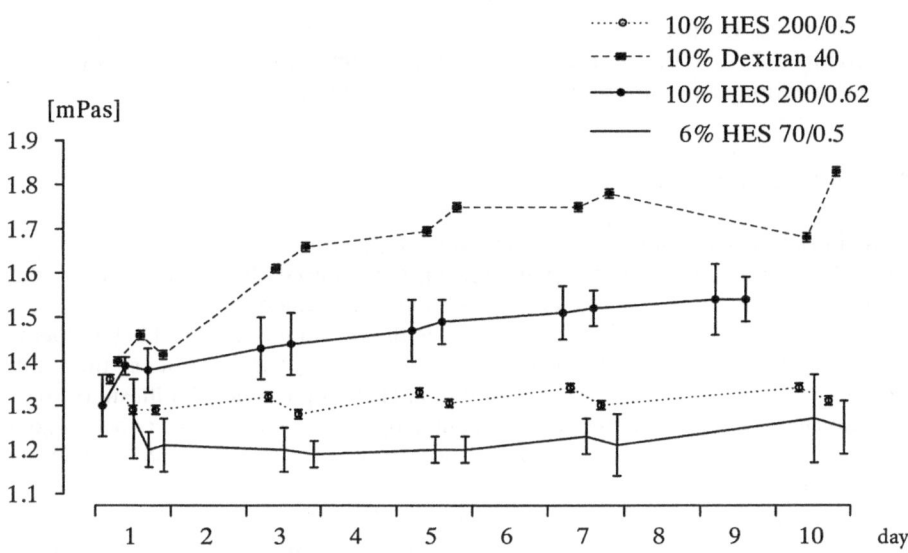

Fig. 4. Effect of a long-term infusion of 10% HES 200/0.5, 10% Dextran 40, 10% HES 200/0.62 and 6% HES 70/0.5 on plasma viscosity

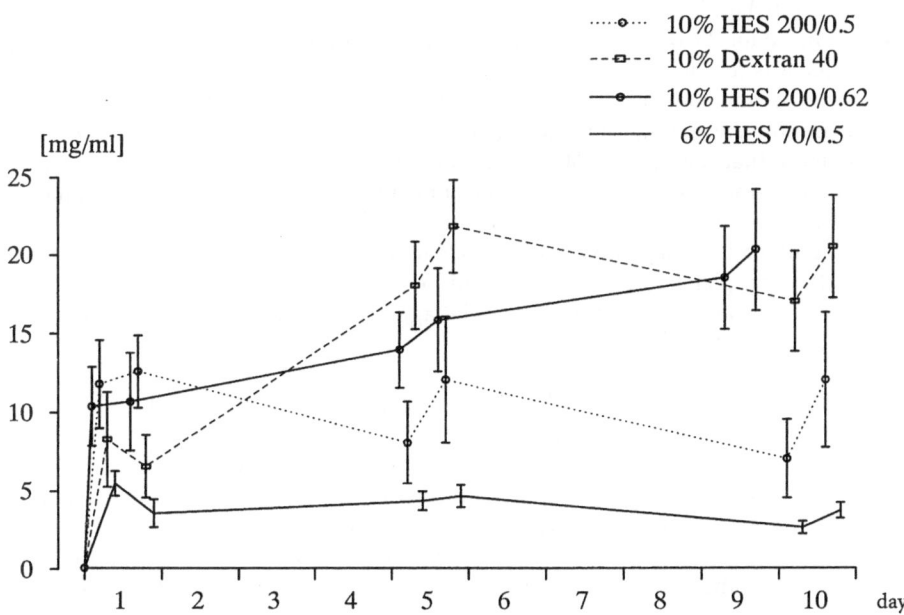

Fig. 5. Serum concentration of 10% HES 200/0.5, 10% Dextran 40, 10% HES 200/0.62 and 6% HES 70/0.5 after a long-term infusion therapy

was observed. The measured concentrations were for medium molecular weight starch approximately 10 mg/ml. For the low molecular weight starch which was only infused as 6% solution, the values ranged from 2.6 to 5.4 mg/ml.

Hemostasiological Parameters

The initial platelet count was very similar for all groups at the beginning, ranging from 237,000 to 246,000/mm^3 (Fig. 6). No group showed changes beyond the dilution effect, which can be judged from the change in hematocrit.

The initial values of the patients treated with HES 200/0.62 ranged before therapy from 173,000 to 328,000/mm^3. Mean value was 240,700±55.600/mm^3. Before the last day of infusion, the lowest value was 194,000/mm^3. This drop was not significant (p>0.05). In the Dextran 40 group, the platelet count dropped on day 1 from 244,000±43,000/mm^3 to 206,000±43,000/mm^3. On day 10, the value was 202,000±35,000/mm^3. HES 200/0.5 lowered the platelet count during the 10-day therapy from 246,000 ±69,000/mm^3 to 243,000±34,000/mm^3. In the group treated with low molecular weight starch, platelet count was before therapy 237,000±40,000/mm^3. The lowest value in this group was reached immediately after the loading dose at 217,000±40,000/mm^3. During the remaining infusion therapy, platelet number increased again and was on day 10 higher (261,000±41,000/mm^3) than the initial value.

During the infusion therapy with HES 200/0.5 (1) a slight decrease of *mean platelet volume* (Fig. 7) from 10.29±1.07 μm^3 to 9.8 μm^3 was observed. Infusion of HES 70/0.5 resulted in a decrease from 10.36±1.25 μm^3 to 9.88 μm^3. This decrease was significant (p<0.05) for both substances with the exception of day 3. The decrease was more pronounced for the 0.62 substituted starch. Initial volume was 9.67±2.16 μm^3, the lowest value was reached on day 7 at 8.43 μm^3 (-12.8%, significant).

Dextrans and and HES have different effects on *platelet aggregation*. Whereas Dextrans inhibit the spontanous and induced platelet aggregation, HES 200/0.62 is the only starch that causes a slight decrease in platelet aggregation. The alpha2-angle of the rotation-induced spontaneous platelet aggregation was lowered through the volume therapy with HES 200/0.62 from 30.7°±25.6° to 14.2°±18.2°. This decrease was only significiant on day 5 and 7 (p<0.05). For HES 200/0.5 and HES 70/0.5 no significant effect on platelet aggregation could be observed. For the low molecular HES, the alpha-2-angle of spontaneous platelet aggregation was on day 10 above the initial value (22.2°±15.4° vs. 11.9°± 13.9°).

The infusion of the loading dose of HES 200/0.5 resulted in a small decline of the *quick* value from 87.5±12.6% to 86.7% (Fig. 8). During the remaining therapy, the quick fluctuated little and was at the end of therapy at 89.0% slightly above the initial value. The first Dextran infusion lead to a significant decrease (p<0.05), leading to an overall drop at the end of day 1 from 93%±6% to 77%. The quick on the last day was 72%. The reduction in quick was therefore most pronounced in the Dextran group, followed by the 0.62 substituted HES, which caused a 20% drop from the initial value (99.3%±1.0%).

HES 70/0.5 and HES 200/0.5 caused no changes in quick. Initial value was 99.1%±2.7%, the maximum decrease 8.5% (n.s.).

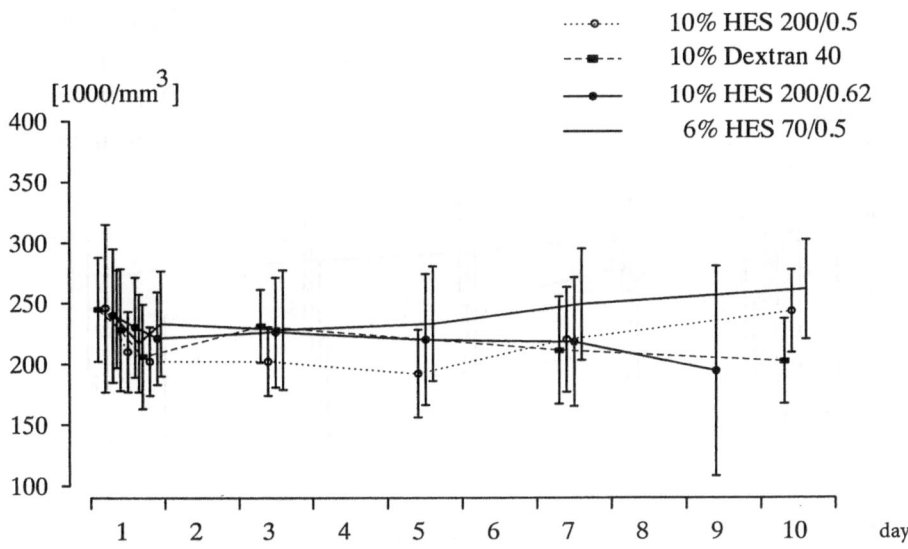

Fig. 6. Effect of a long-term infusion of 10% HES 200/0.5, 10% Dextran 40, 10% HES 200/0.62 and 6% HES 70/0.5 on platelet count

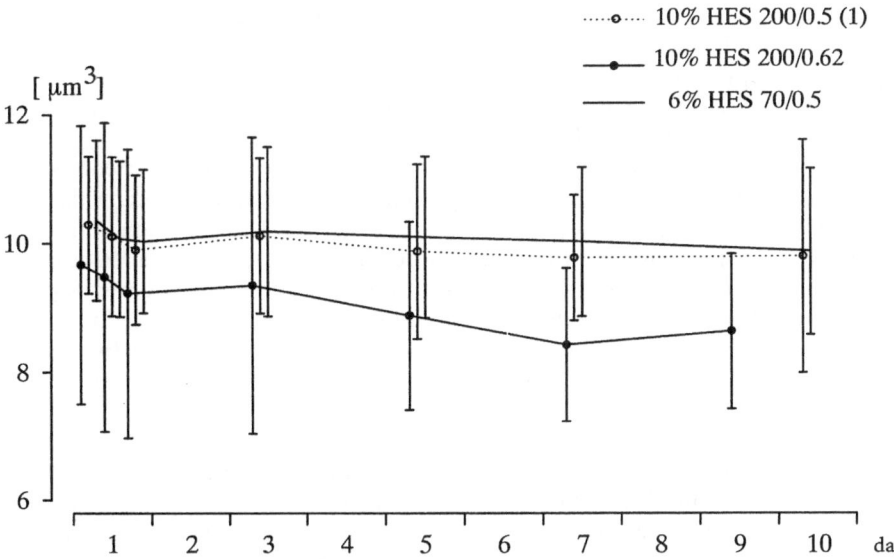

Fig. 7. Effect of a long-term infusion of 10% HES 200/0.5, 10% HES 200/0.62 and 6% HES 70/0.5 on mean platelet volume

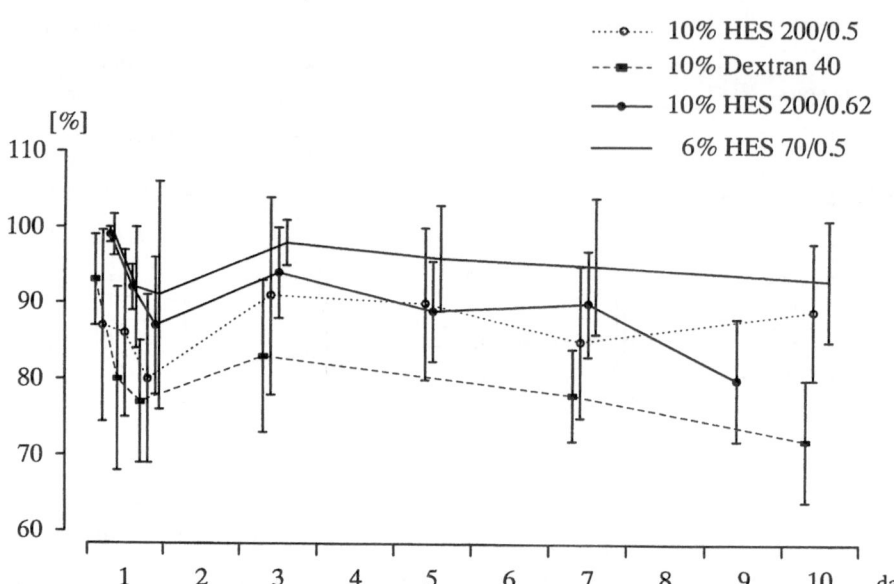

Fig. 8. Effect of a long-term infusion of 10% HES 200/0.5, 10% Dextran 40, 10% HES 200/0.62 and 6% HES 70/0.5 on thromoplastin time (Quick)

HES 200/0.5 caused a 10.8% increase in *PTT* from 36.7±3.4 s to 40.7±5.9 s (Fig. 9). Dextran raised the initial value (32.2±1.6 s) by 23.9% to 39.9±2.0 s. The higher substituted HES 200/0.62 increased PTT by 42.8%. The initial value was 29.9±0.9 s and was increased by the loading dose significantly to 31.7%±1.9 s and increased further during therapy to 42.7±3.3 s. In the low molecular weight HES group PTT was initially 32.1±1.2 s. This particular plasma substitute had no significant effect on PTT. The final PTT was only 4% above the initial value (33.4±2.4 s).

At the beginning of therapy, the rapid infusion of HES 200/0.5 shortened *thrombin time* from 19.6±2.0 s to 17.7 s (Fig. 10). During the remaining therapy, thrombin time hardly changed, final value on day 10 was 18.4±1.2 s. The reduction in thrombin time was more pronounced for Dextran. The loading dose caused an 28.2% drop from the initial value of 20.6±0.5 s. At the end of therapy, thrombin time was 15.5±1.1 s, corresponding to a 24.7% drop. The rapid infusion of HES 200/0.62 led to a 28.9% decrease from the initial value of 22.8±11.1 s, and a further significant (p<0.05) decline to 13.7%±1.1 s during the remaining therapy. Low molecular weight HES caused only small changes in thrombin time, which dropped at the end of therapy from 17.3±1.1 s 16.4±0.9 s.

Figure 11 shows the effect of the different plasma substitutes on *fibrinogen concentration*. A loading dose of HES 200/0.5 lowered fibrinogen concentration by 19.9% from 355±82.6 mg% to 284 mg%. During the remainder of therapy, only small changes were observed. The Dextran group showed a very similar initial concentration (349±62 mg%). Under therapy with Dextran, a continuous, 34.7% decrease down to 228 mg% was observed. The first infusion of the highly substituted starch caused a

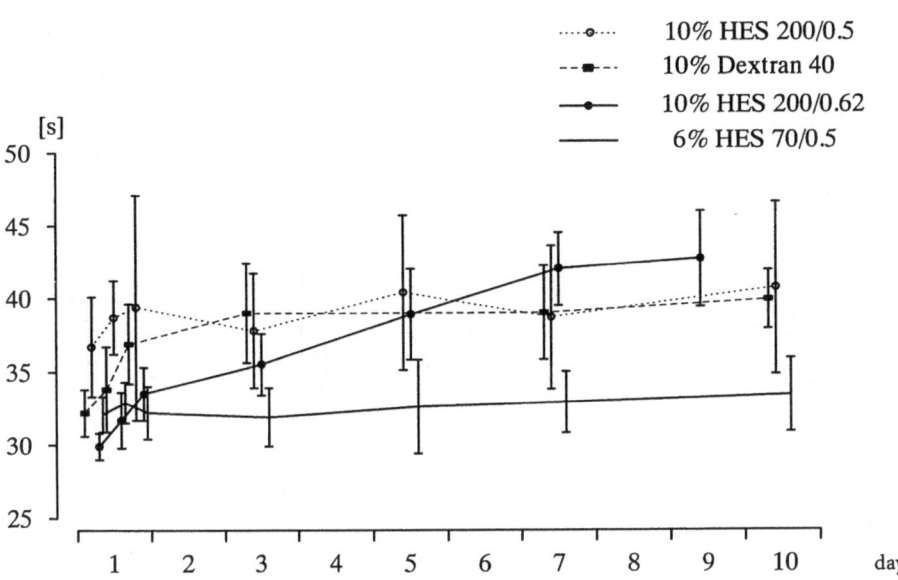

Fig. 9. Effect of a long-term infusion of 10% HES 200/0.5, 10% Dextran 40, 10% HES 200/0.62 and 6% HES 70/0.5 on PTT

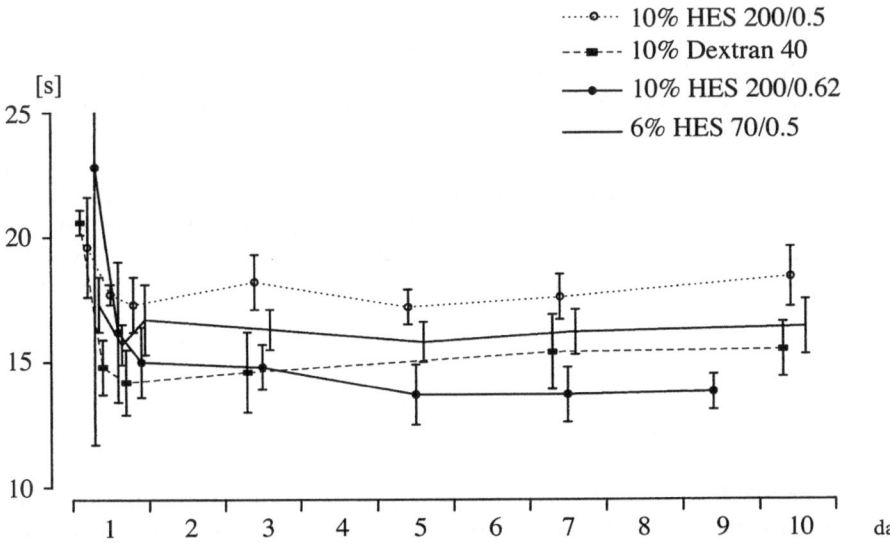

Fig. 10. Effect of a long-term infusion of 10% HES 200/0.5, 10% Dextran 40, 10% HES 200/0.62 and 6% HES 70/0.5 on thrombin time

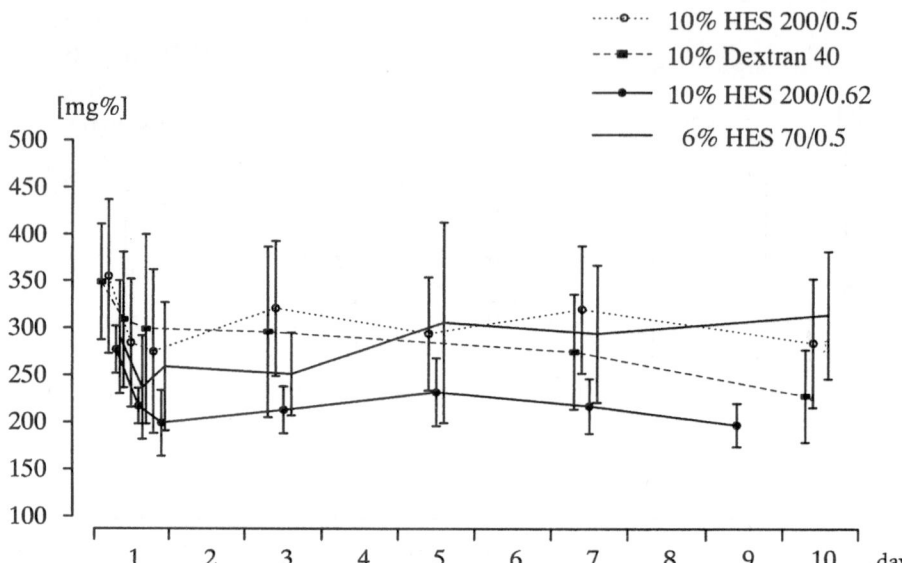

Fig. 11. Effect of a long-term infusion of 10% HES 200/0.5, 10% Dextran 40, 10% HES 200/0.62 and 6% HES 70/0.5 on fibrinogen concentration

decrease in fibrinogen from 278±25 mg% to 217 mg%. Later infusions caused no notable changes. The low molecular weight HES caused the greatest drop from the initial value after the loading dose, 18.2% below the initial concentration (290± 60 mg%). The highest value was measured on day 10 at 315 mg%, which was higher than the initial value.

Long-term infusion of HES 200/0.5 (1) (degree of substitution 13.4) caused a significant ($p < 0.01$) decrease in *coagulation factor II* (prothrombin) from 99.6±16.2% to 69.2±11.2%. HES 70/0.5 lowered this factor through the loading dose significantly ($p < 0.01$) from 107.2±16.3% to 90.4±17.0% ($p < 0.01$). During the remaining therapy, the concentration increased slightly and reached 101.2±17.5% on day 10.

Initial *factor V* concentration in the HES 200/0.5 (1) group was 59.9±19.7%. The lowest value was reached on day 3 at 41.5±16.1% (30.7% below the initial value). In the group treated with low molecular weight HES, lowest factor V activity was observed at the end of day one, 20.3% below the initial value (down to 54.8±17.7% from initial 68.8±14.2%).

HES 200/0.5 (1) lowered *factor VII* during the rapid infusion from 83.5±23.7% to 56.7±16.7% ($p < 0.01$). During therapy, the concentration of factor V reached 69.4±14.8% on day 10. HES 70/0.5 also caused the greatest drop directly after the rapid infusion (68.1±22.0%). This was a significant ($p < 0.01$) 21.6% decrease from the initial activity (86.9±25.9%).

Factor VIII:C was affected very differently by the different plasma substitutes (Fig. 12). The loading dose of 0.5 substituted HES with an initial molecuar weight of 200,000 D caused only a small decrease in factor VIII:C activity from 120.4±53.7% to 109.6%. During the remaining therapy, only small changes occurred, the final value

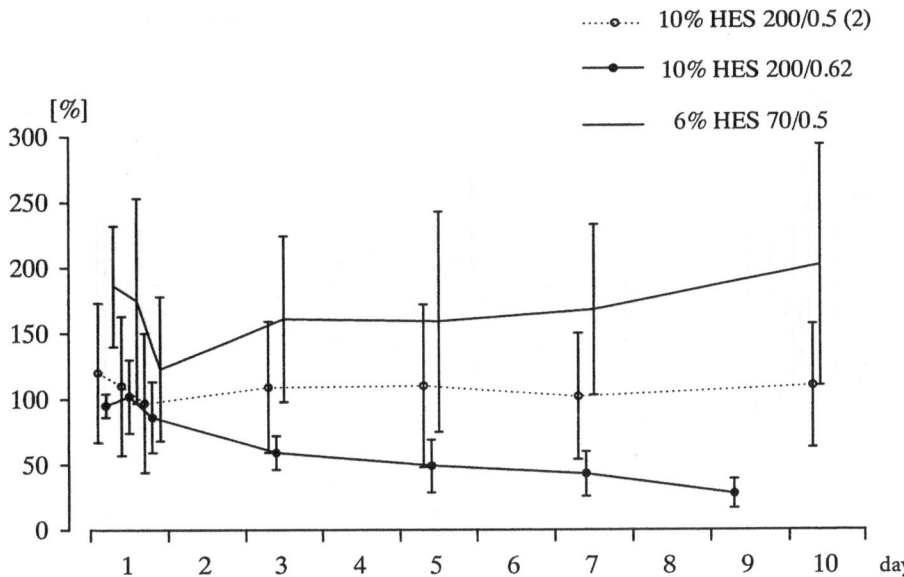

Fig. 12. Effect of a long-term infusion of 10% HES 200/0.5, 10% HES 200/0.62 and 6% HES 70/0.5 on factor VIII:C activity

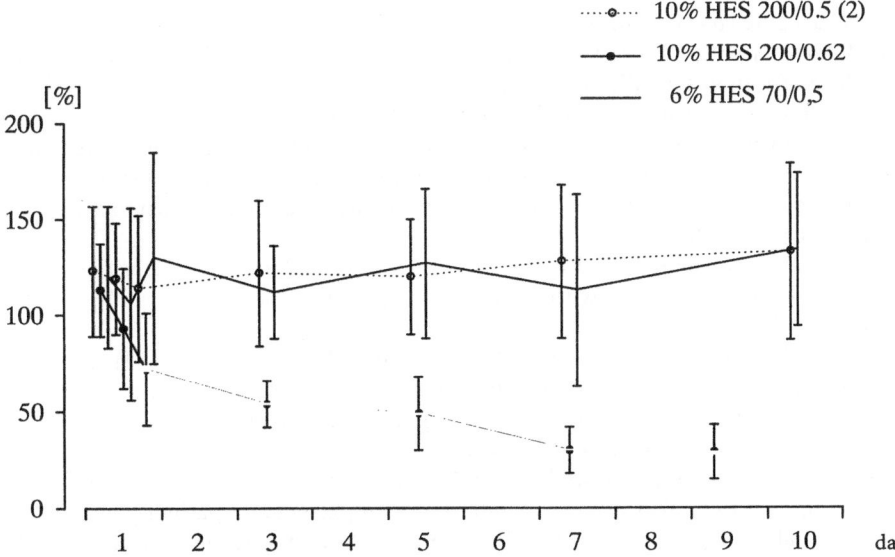

Fig. 13. Effect of a long-term infusion of 10% HES 200/0.5, 10% HES 200/0.62 and 6% HES 70/0.5 on von Willebrand Ristocetin Cofactor

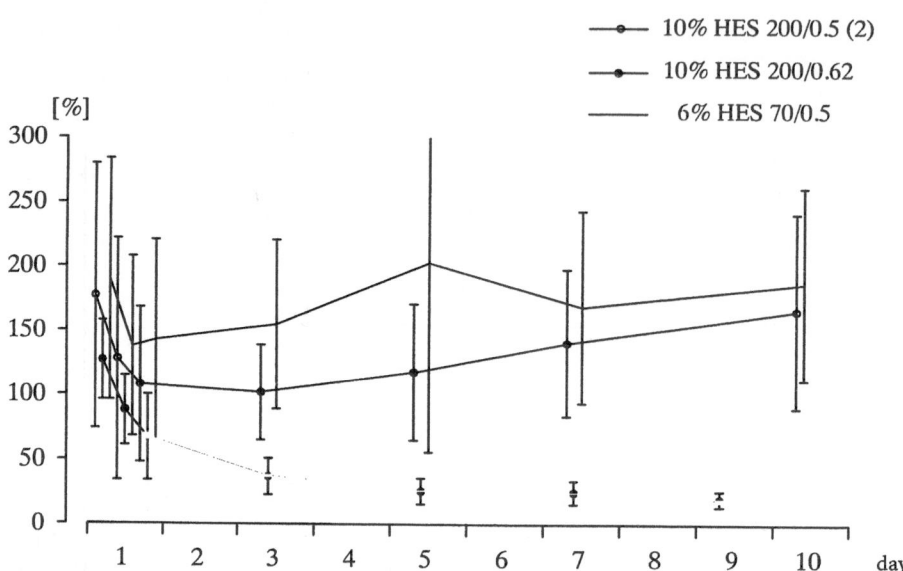

Fig. 14. Effect of a long-term infusion of 10% HES 200/0.5, 10% HES 200/0.62 and 6% HES 70/0.5 on von Willebrand factor antigen

was 110.9%. The more highly substituted starch on the other hand caused a significant decrease to 28.3% (-70.5%). Low molecular HES caused a significant decrease in factor VIII:C activity only at the end of day 1 (down to 123.3% from 186.6±46.9%). Factor VIII:C was not lowered significantly during the remaining time, activity on day 10 was even higher than the initial activity (202.0%).

Measuring *von Willebrand Ristocetin cofactor* yielded comparable results (Fig. 13). HES 200/0.5 with a more favorable substitution pattern (C2/C6 ratio 5.7) and low molecular weight HES did not siginificantly affect von Willebrand Ristocetin cofactor. Activities measured during infusion therapy changed a maximum of 12% from the initial values (123.0±34.0% and 120.4±37.5%, respectively) and were at the end of therapy even higher than the initial values. However, similar to factor VIII:C, the more highly (0.62) substituted HES caused a 70% decrease in activity (down to 29.7±14.7% from 113.3±24.1%).

Similar to von Willebrand Ristocetin cofactor, *von Willebrand factor antigen* was affected little by a therapy with HES 200/0.5 and HES 70/0.5 (Fig. 14). Medium molecular weight HES 200/0.5 caused a drop from 177±103.7% to 102.7%, low molecular weight HES from 190.9±94.1% to 138.7%. The more highly substituted HES 200/0.62 led directly after the initial infusion to a significant decrease from 127.5±31.9% to 88.3%. Von Willebrand factor antigen dropped continuously until the last day of infusions to 20.8±6.6% (84.4% below the initial value). A control analysis 3 to 4 days after the end of therapy showed a slight increase to 26.8%.

Compared to pooled plasma, standard human plasma and patient plasma before therapy, all patients treated with HES 200/0.62 showed a decrease in the complete multimer spectrum of von Willebrand factor after the beginning of therapy (Fig. 15). The decrease continued during therapy, all multimers were still present. Because all

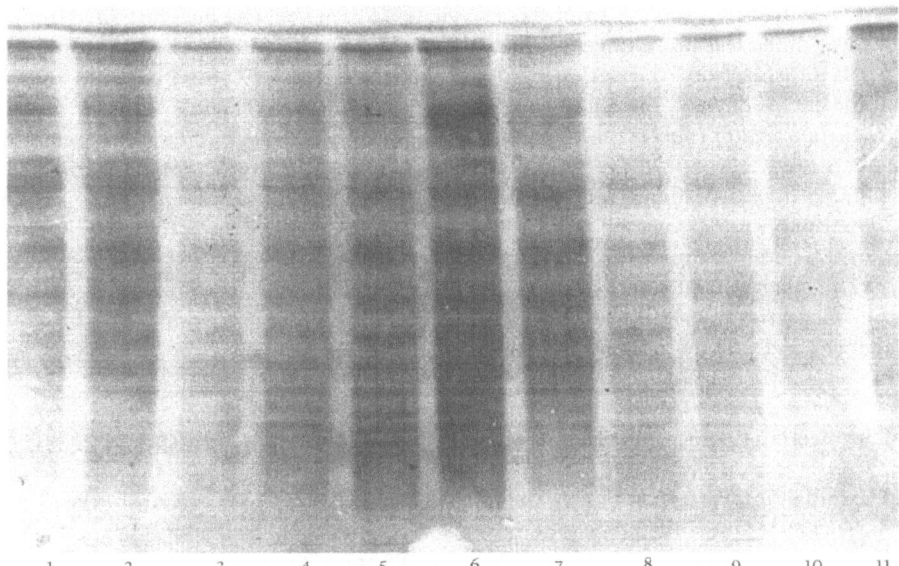

Fig. 15. Analysis of von Willebrand Factor multimers with SDS agarose gel electrophoresis during a long-term infusion therapy with 10% HES 200/0.62 in 2 patients: 1: pool plasma; 2: patient A before infusion therapy; 3: patient A, day 5; 4: patient A day 10; 5: patient A day 13; 6: standard human plasma; 7: patient B before infusion; 8: patient B day 5; 9: patient B day 10; 10: patient B day 13; 11: standard human plasma

multimers were affected similarly, the observed decrease was most likely a purely quantitative effect. This corresponds to an acquired (type 1) von Willebrand syndrome (Holmberg and Nilsson 1985, Rugeri 1994).

Factor IX was not lowered significantly by HES 200/0.5 (1) or HES 70/0.5, with both starches causing the greatest drop during the high-dose phase. The rapid infusion of HES 200/0.5 (1) lowered the activity of factor IX from 109.7±25.7% to 84.5±17.9%. In the following days, mean values ranged from 92.1% to 96.2%. The initial value in the HES 70/0.5 group was 116.0±30.5%, decreased until day 3 to 95.8±18.5% and increased again in the following days, reaching a final value on the last day above the initial activity (126.0±53.6%).

Factor X (Stuart-Prower factor) was lowered significantly (p<0.01) by HES 200/0.5 from 87.6±14.3% to 59.8±8.7% (-13%). Low molecular weight HES caused only a 17.8% drop (from 90.1±18.2% to 74.0±15.8%). For HES 200/0.5 (1), the decrease was greatest on day 5, for HES 70/0.5 on day 3. After the end of the high-dose infusion period, factor X increased slowly in both groups.

Activity of *factor XI* was reduced by 49.0% through infusion of HES 200/0.62 (from 104.8±16.6% to 53.4±7.8%). Three days after the end of volume therapy, factor XI activity increased again to 62.4±10.6%. The effect of HES 200/0.5 (1) and HES 70/0.5 on factor XI was smaller. HES 200 caused a drop from 93.7±21.2% to 52.4±9.9%, while HES 70 lowered factor XI from 87.9±17.2% to 74.3±14.2%.

For the highly substituted HES (200/0.62), the reduction in *factor XII* activity was similar to factor XI (from 98.7% to 53.7%). HES 200/0.5 decreased activity of factor

XII significantly (p<0.01) from 67.5±21.5% to 40.8±9.5%. The decrease for HES 70/0.5 was much less pronounced. Activity decreased significantly (p<0.05) through the rapid infusion from 71.4±24.3% before therapy to 59.8±20.1%, but increased already at the end of day 1.

C1-inactivator concentration and *-activity* were only measured for the more highly substituted HES 200/0.62. The initial value of C1-inactivator concentration was 28.1±5.8 mg%, the final value on the last day 29.4 mg%. Initial activity of the C1-inactivator was on average 86.0±15.5%. Until the end of day 1, activity declined to 69.7%. There were no significant changes in C1-inactivator concentration or activity.

The measurements of thrombin/antithrombin III-complex carried out in the HES 200/0.62 group also showed no significant changes and were 3.6±2.1 µg/l before therapy and 3.9±2.9 µg/l on the last day.

Fibronectin, Amylase, Lipase, and Blood Count

The initial *fibronectin concentration* in the HES 200/0.62 group ranged from 13.5 to 42.0 mg% (Fig. 16), mean value was 26.0±9.1%. All patients showed a significant drop in fibronectin concentration (p<0.01). The 10% HES 200/0.62 group showed a continuous, 62.4% drop until day 13, from 26.6±9.2 mg% to 10.0±2.2 mg%. One patient showed a clinically asymptomatic drop from 41.0 down to 6.4%. The group treated with 6% HES 200/0.62 showed a continuous decrease from 25.5±9.9% to 15.0±3.2 mg% on day 10.

Long-term therapy with HES 200/0.62 resulted in a significant (p<0.05), more than five-fold increase of *alpha-amylases* from 75±18.4 U/l to 392. After the end of infu-

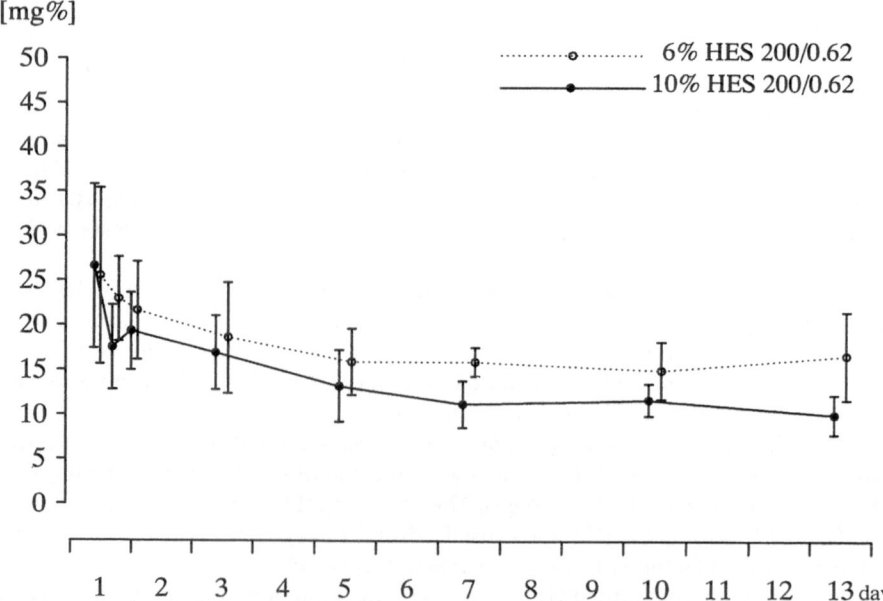

Fig. 16. Effect of a long-term infusion therapy with 6% and 10% HES 200/0.62 on fibronectin

sions, alpha-amylases returned to normal slowly, on day 13 alpha-amylase concentration was still at 351.8 U/l.

Lipase activity in the serum was not affected considerably. Long-term infusion of HES 200/0.62 caused a slight decrease from 96.9±22.1 U/l to 71.8 U/l.

As expected, the *blood count* showed a dilution-induced significant (p<0.01) decline in erythrocyte number and hemoglobin concentration. HES 200/0.5 (1) reduced *erythrocyte count* from 4.95±0.22×10⁶/µl to 3.67×10⁶/µl, HES 70/0.5 caused a reduction from 4.93±0.24×10⁶/µl to 4.08×10⁶/µl. *Hemoglobin concentration* decreased from 15.7±0.5 g/dl to 11.9 g/dl in the group with medium molecular weight HES. Low molecular weight HES caused only a small decrease from 15.6±0.7 g/dl to 13.0 g/dl. Initial *mean corpuscular hemoglobin* was 31.8±1.4 pg for HES 200/0.5 (1) and did not change significantly during the therapy, reaching an almost identical value on day 10 (31.9±1.0). In the control group, the initial value was 31.6±1.3 pg, the final value 32.0±1.1 pg. Patients treated with HES 200/0.5 (1) also showed no significant changes in *mean corpuscular hemoglobin concentration*, with an initial value of 34.1±0.7 and a final value of 34.0±0.6. For the low molecular weight HES, initial and final values were similar at 34.6±0.92 and 35.2±0.7, respectively. Mean corpuscular volume of the erythrocytes showed a small, yet significant (p<0.01) decrease: from 93.1±4.2 fl to 92.5±4.1 fl in the HES 200/0.5 (1) group and from 91.3±4.0 to 90.7±3.8 in the HES 70/0.5 group. *Volume distribution width* also decreased minimally in both groups. Medium molecular weight HES caused a decrease from 12.0±0.8 to 11.8±0.9 on day 1 (p<0.05), low molecular weight HES a decrese from 12.0±1.0 to 11.6±1.1% (p<0.01). *Leukocyte count* dropped in the HES 200/0.5 (1) group immediately after the loading dose from 8,600±4,600/µl to 7,000±3,500/µl (p<0.01) and increased afterwards, reaching the initial number. The initial count in the other group was 6,600±1,600 and did not change significantly during the therapy. The percentage of *lymphocytes* dropped significantly in both groups (p<0.01). Medium molecular weight HES caused a drop in the percentage from 28.6±11.3% to 19.6±7.7%, low molecular weight HES a drop from 33.8±7.7% to 29.4±7.9%. The share of *neutrophilic granulocytes* increased in both groups significantly (p<0.02), with an increase from 58.9±14.1% to 69.1±10.0% in the HES 200/0.5 (1) group and an increase from 54.6±8.8% to 59.3±8.5% in the HES 70/0.5 group.

Influence of the HES Substitution Pattern

We studied the effect of the substitution pattern with two 10% HES 200/0.5 solutions that were identical except for their C2/C6 substitution pattern. In the following, they are called 10% HES 200/0.5 (1) and (2). HES 200/0.5 (1) has a C2/C6 ratio of 13.4 and HES 200/0.5 (2) a C2/C6 ratio of 5.7. According to animal studies by Yoshida et al. (1973 and 1984), it is to be expected that HES 200/0.5 (1) with the higher C2/C6 ratio of 13.4, i.e. a higher share of hydroxyethyl substitution at carbon 2 is metabolized more slowly.

Figure 17 shows the effects of the different substitution patterns on *hematocrit*. Initial hematocrit in the HES (1) group was higher than in the HES (2) group (47.2% vs. 42.9%, respectively). Bloodletting and loading dose caused an 18% decrease in both groups. The lowest value of 32.8% was reached in group 1 on day 7 and in group 2 on day 5. This corresponds to a 30.5% and 23.5% drop, respectively. HES 200/0.5 (1) has a stronger dilution effect, which occurs however with a delay.

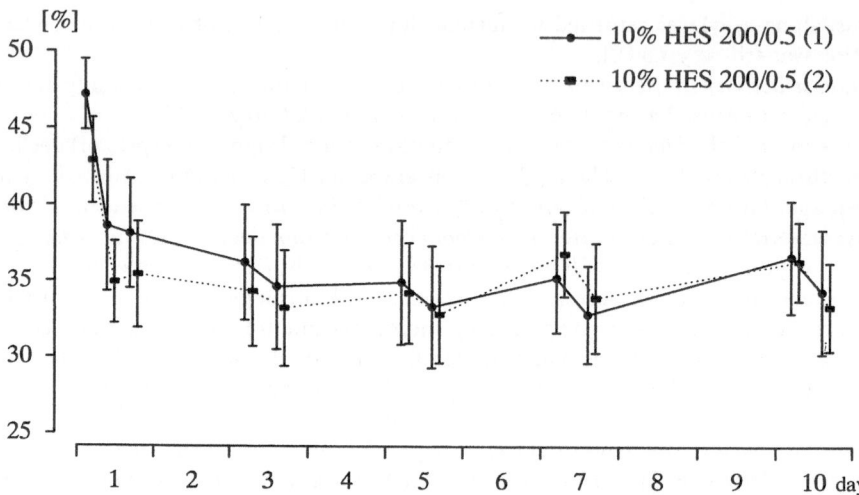

Fig. 17. Effect of a long-term infusion therapy with two different 10% HES 200/0.5 solutions with differing C2/C6 hydroxyethylation ratios on hematocrit. The C2/C6 hydroxyethylation ratio for HES 200/0.5 (1) was 13.4 and for HES 200/0.5 (2) it was 5.7 (modified from Treib et al. 1995)

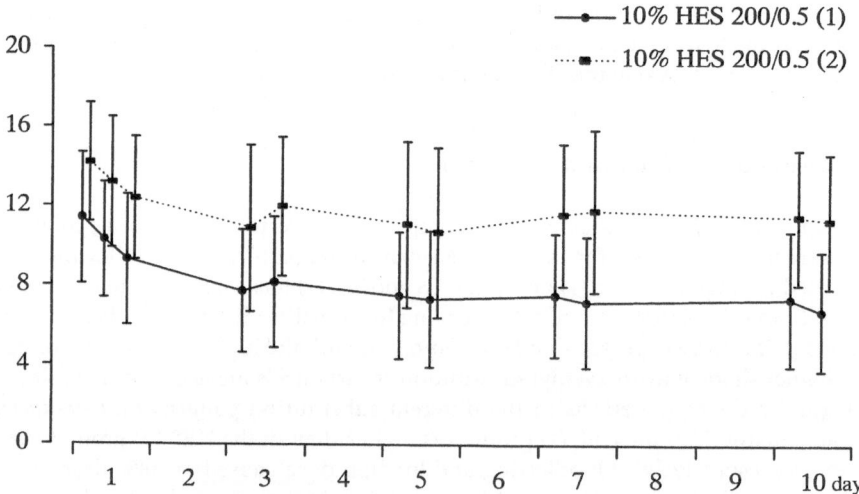

Fig. 18. Effect of a long-term infusion therapy with two different 10% HES 200/0.5 solutions with differing C2/C6 hydroxyethylation ratios on erythrocyte aggregation. The C2/C6 hydroxyethylation ratio for HES 200/0.5 (1) was 13.4 and for HES 200/0.5 (2) it was 5.7 (modified from Treib et al. 1995)

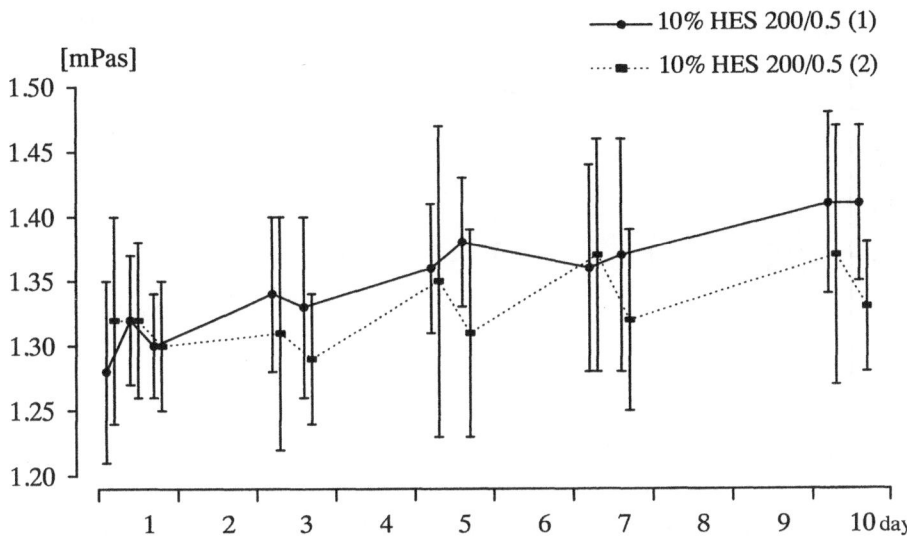

Fig. 19. Effect of a long-term infusion therapy with two different 10% HES 200/0.5 solutions with differing C2/C6 hydroxyethylation ratios on plasma viscosity. The C2/C6 hydroxyethylation ratio for HES 200/0.5 (1) was 13.4 and for HES 200/0.5 (2) it was 5.7 (modified from Treib et al. 1995)

Erythrocyte aggregation (Fig. 18) was before therapy lower in group 1 (11.4±3.3) than in group 2 (14.2±3.0). In both groups, a lower tendency to aggregate was observed, with a higher maximum in group 1 (41%) than in group 2 (24.6%).

Figure 19 shows that the starch with a higher C2/C6 ratio caused a continuous, significant ($p<0.05$) 10% increase in *plasma viscosity* (from 1.28±0.07 mPas to 1.41±0.07 mPas). HES (2) on the other hand caused a smaller increase (4%), starting on day 5 (from 1.32±0.08 mPas to 1.37±0.10 mPas).

The measurements of *serum concentration* (Fig. 20) of HES 200/0.5 (1) showed in the high-dose phase a continuous increase (from 9.3±1.1 mg/ml to 14.9±1.0 mg/ml). In the following low-dose phase, concentration decreased again to 12.0 mg/ml. The starch solution with the low C2/C6 ratio of 5.7 showed no accumulation of HES in the serum. The concentration of 9.0±2.1 mg/ml reached during the loading dose, remained stable during the high-dose infusion therapy and dropped towards the end of therapy to 5.8±1.2 mg/ml.

The effect on *PTT* (Fig. 21) showed a clear dependency on the substitution pattern. Whereas the starch with a high C2/C6 ratio caused a significant, 30% increase in PTT (from 31.2±2.3 s to 40.6±4.4 s), the PTT increase was much smaller in the other group (13%, from 30.2±2.9 s to 34.0±3.0 s).

Thromboplastin time (quick) was not considerably affected by either substance. Initial values were closely together (92.3±8.6% for HES (1) and 95.3±7.4% for HES (2)). Reduction in quick was 11.9% in group 1 and 6.1% in group 2.

The shortening of *thrombin time* was also more pronounced in group 1 than in group 2 (24.0% vs. 16.6%, respectively). Initial values were comparable in both groups (17.5±1.28 s vs. 16.2±0.6 s).

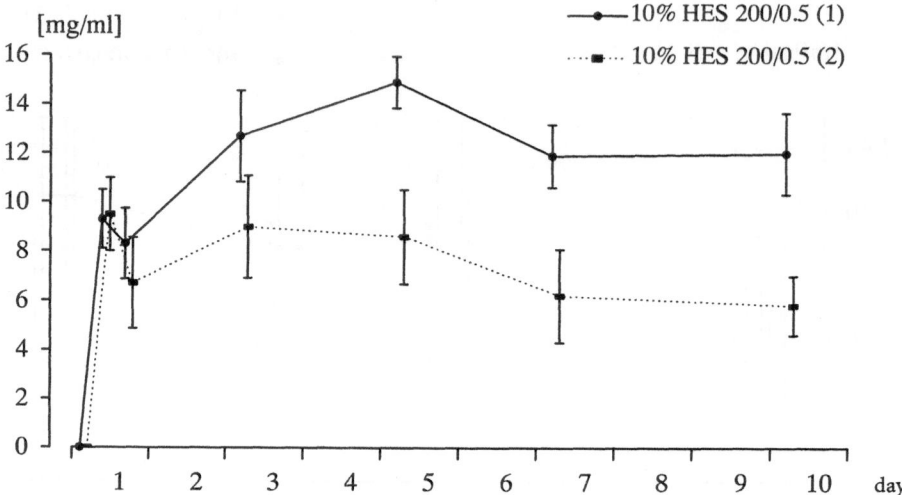

Fig. 20. Effect of a long-term infusion therapy with two different 10% HES 200/0.5 solutions with differing C2/C6 hydroxyethylation ratios on HES serum concentration. The C2/C6 hydroxyethylation ratio for HES 200/0.5 (1) was 13.4 and for HES 200/0.5 (2) it was 5.7 (modified from Treib et al. 1995)

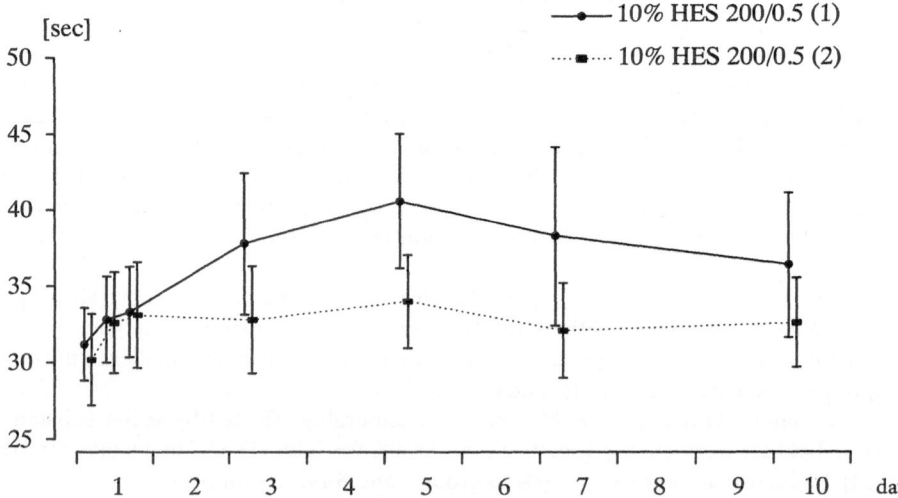

Fig. 21. Effect of a long-term infusion therapy with two different 10% HES 200/0.5 solutions with differing C2/C6 hydroxyethylation ratios on PTT. The C2/C6 hydroxyethylation ratio for HES 200/0.5 (1) was 13.4 and for HES 200/0.5 (2) it was 5.7 (modified from Treib et al. 1995)

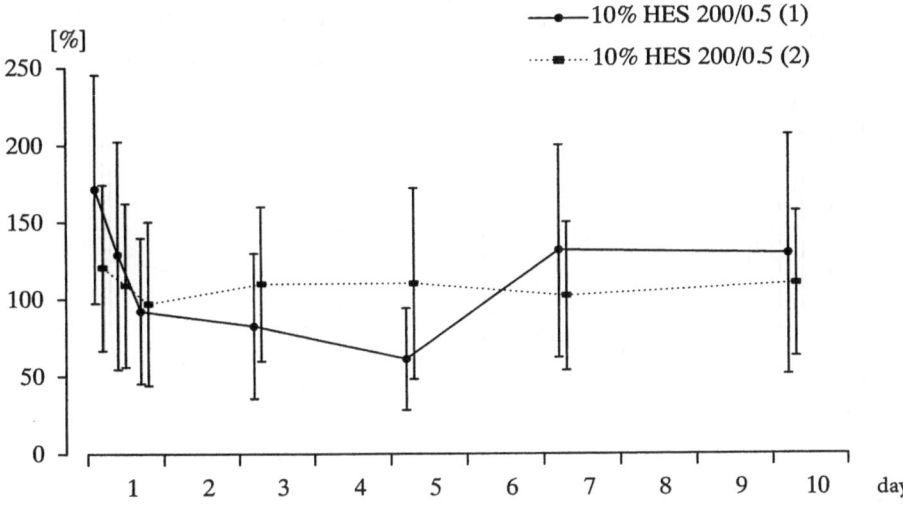

Fig. 22. Effect of a long-term infusion therapy with two different 10% HES 200/0.5 solutions with differing C2/C6 hydroxyethylation ratios on factor VIII:C. The C2/C6 hydroxyethylation ratio for HES 200/0.5 (1) was 13.4 and for HES 200/0.5 (2) it was 5.7 (modified from Treib et al. 1995)

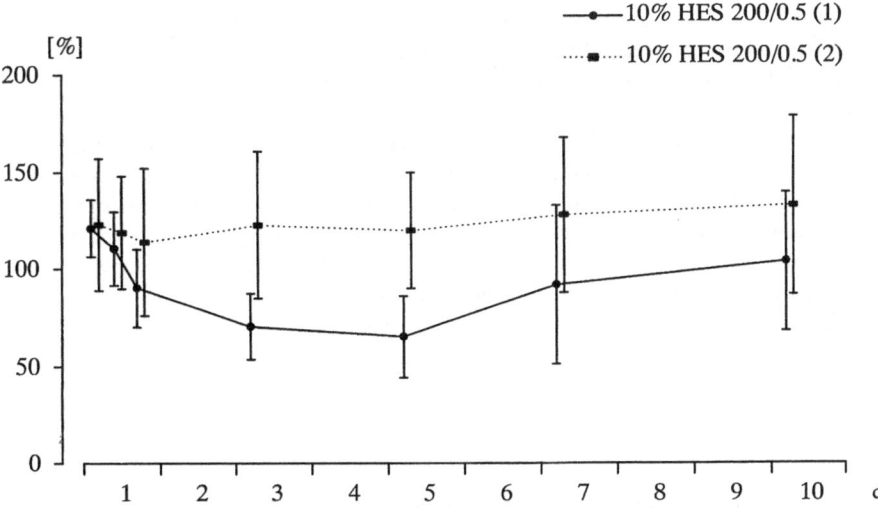

Fig. 23. Effect of a long-term infusion therapy with two different 10% HES 200/0.5 solutions with differing C2/C6 hydroxyethylation ratios on von Willebrand Ristocetin co-factor. The C2/C6 hydroxyethylation ratio for HES 200/0.5 (1) was 13.4 and for HES 200/0.5 (2) it was 5.7 (modified from Treib et al. 1995)

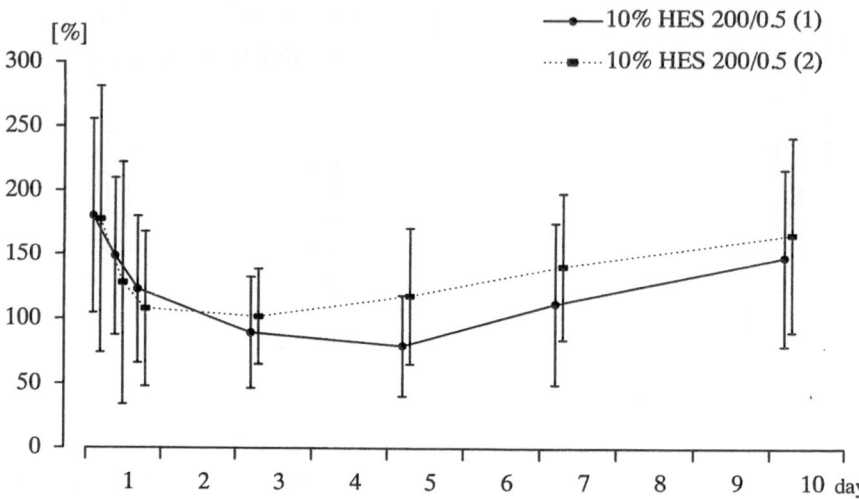

Fig. 24. Effect of a long-term infusion therapy with two different 10% HES 200/0.5 solutions with differing C2/C6 hydroxyethylation ratios on von Willebrand factor antigen. The C2/C6 hydroxyethylation ratio for HES 200/0.5 (1) was 13.4 and for HES 200/0.5 (2) it was 5.7 (modified from Treib et al. 1995)

Fibrinogen concentration decreased by 29.0% (p<0.01, from 292.6±111.2 mg%) in group 1 and by 25.0% (p<0.01, from 239.3±77.8) in group 2.

The most pronounced difference between the two HES solutions was observed in their effect on factor VIII/von Willebrand factor complex. HES 200/0.5 (1), which is degraded more slowly due to its higher C2/C6 ratio of 13.4, reduced *factor VIII:C* (Fig. 22) strongly (from 171.5±74.0% to 61.2±32.9%). The starch with the lower C2/C6 ratio of 5.7 caused a much smaller decline of 19.3% (120.4±53.6% to 97.1±53.7%).

Under therapy with HES 200/0.5 (1) *von Willebrand Ristocetin Cofactor* decreased by 45.6% (down from 121.1±14.8%, Fig. 23), the lowest value was reached on day 5 at 65.9±20.2%. The decrease in group 2 was only 7%. HES 200/0.5 (2) lowered von Willebrand Ristocetin Cofactor at the end of day 1 from 123.0±34.0 to 114.3±38.0%. During the remaining therapy, von Willebrand Ristocetin co-factor increased again and the final value was higher then the initial activity (134.4±409%).

The decrease in *von Willebrand factor antigen* (Fig. 24) was also larger in group 1 (55.8%) than in group 2 (42.2%). Under therapy with HES 200/0.5 (1) von Willebrand factor antigen decreased from 180.2±75.5% to 79.7±38.4%, under HES 200/0.5 (2) the decrease was smaller (177.6±103.7% to 102.7±37.2%).

Distribution of the Molecular Weight of HES

The examination of the distribution of the molecular weight explains the different attributes of the studied HES.

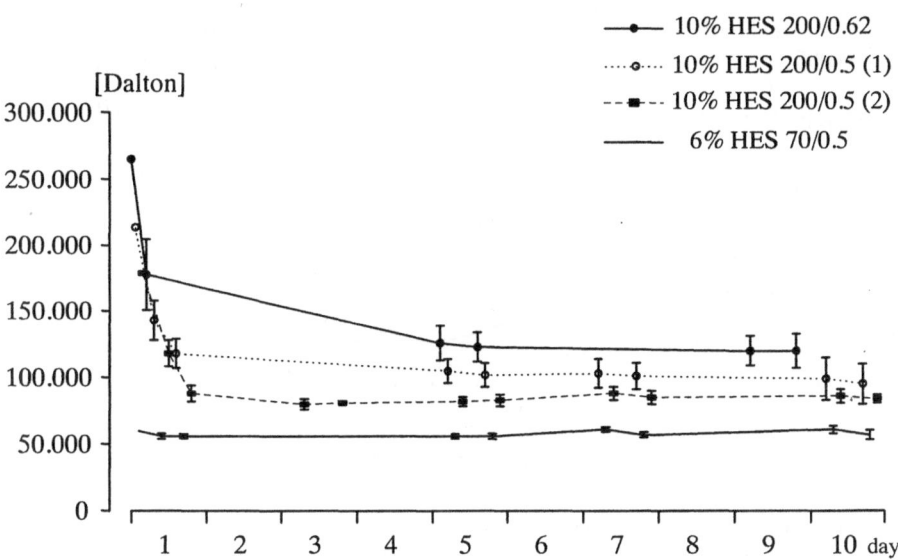

Fig. 25. Weight averaged molecular weight (Mw) of serum starches after a long-term infusion therapy with two different 10% HES 200/0.5 solutions with differing C2/C6 hydroxyethylation ratios, 10% HES 200/0.62 and 6% HES 70/0.5

Figure 25 shows the weight averaged molecular weight (Mw) of the plasma substitutes during the volume therapy. The in-vitro Mw of the HES 200/0.62 infusion solution was 270,000 D. Through rapid enzymatic breakdown, the Mw immediately after the loading dose was reduced to 127,000 D, reaching 120,000 at the end of therapy. HES (1) and (2) had an in-vitro Mw of 214,000 and 180,000 respectively. After the loading dose, the Mw was 144,000 and 118,000 D, respectively, reaching 95,000 and 84,000 on the final day. The low initial Mw of HES 70/0.5 (60,000 D) changed little in vivo, reaching 58,000 D on the last day of therapy.

Due to the more difficult elimination, Dextran leads to an accumulation of larger molecules. The distribution of molecular weight was shifted to the right and a continuous increase from the in-vitro Mw of 52,000 to an in-vivo Mw on the last day of 102,000 was observed. Individual infusions resulted in a short-time lowering of Mw, due to the dilution effect.

The analysis of the average molar masses (Mn) showed different trends for different starch solutions. With HES 200/0.62, a slight increase from 66,000 to 85,000 D occurred. HES 200/0.5 (1) showed a decrease from 93,000 to 65,000 D, whereas HES 200/0.5 (2) caused an 11.5% increase of the in-vitro value of 52,000 D. The in-vivo Mn of low molecular weight starch increased considerably from 24,000 to 51,000 D, suggesting a rapid elimination of small molecules.

A study of the *average Mw of the 10% largest molecules* (Fig. 26) showed that the infusion solution of HES 200/0.62 contains suprisingly large molecules, the in-vitro value was 1,091,000 D. In-vivo, the Mw of the 10% largest molecules declined to 307,000 D. For HES 200/0.5 (1) and (2) the inital values were closely together at 768,000 and 782,000 respectively, reaching 241,000 and 221,000, respectively, under therapy.

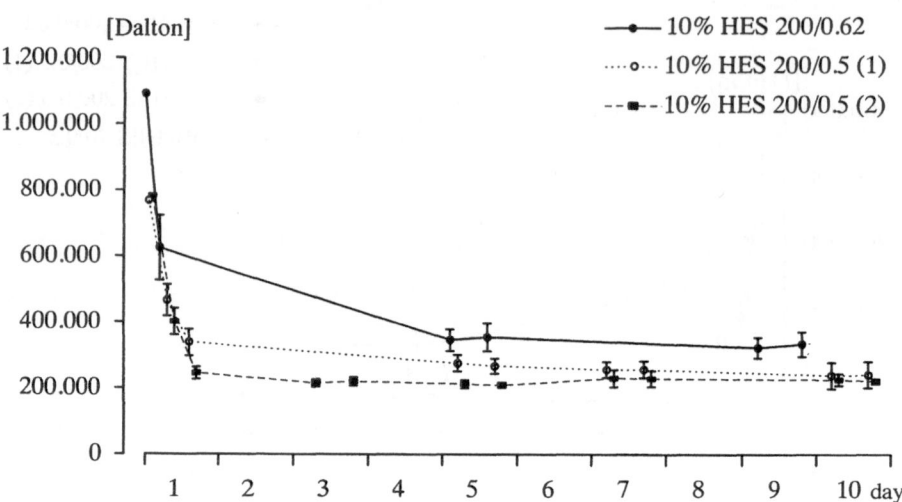

Fig. 26. Average molecular weight (Mw) of the 10% largest molecules of serum starches after a long-term infusion therapy with two different 10% HES 200/0.5 solutions with differing C2/C6 hydroxyethylation ratios, 10% HES 200/0.62 and 6% HES 70/0.5

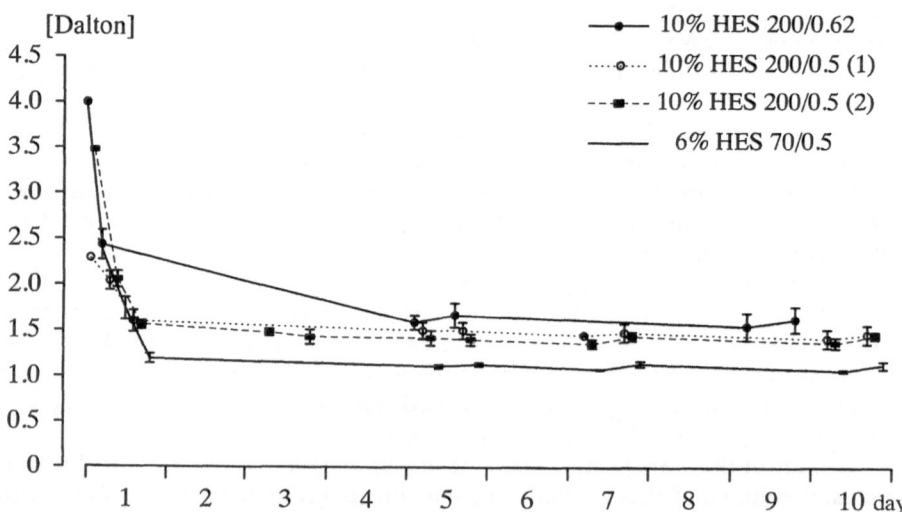

Fig. 27. Width of molecular weight distribution of serum starches after a long-term infusion therapy with two different 10% HES 200/0.5 solutions with differing C2/C6 hydroxyethylation ratios, 10% HES 200/0.62 and 6% HES 70/0.5

The *average Mw of the 10% smallest molecules* showed in the highly substituted HES an in-vitro increase from 18,000 to a maximum of 36,000 D; for HES 200/0.5 (1) it remained constant at 30,000 D, for HES 200/0.5 (2) it increased from 15,000 to 30,000 D.

The *distribution width of the molecular weight* (Fig. 27), indicated by the quotient Mw/Mn narrowed for all starch solution through elimination of the smaller and hydrolysis of the larger molecules. For HES 200/0.62, the quotient dropped rapidly from 4.0 to 1.5. HES 200/0.5 (1) and (2) led to a reduction from 2.3 and 3.5, respectively, to 1.5. Mw/Mn dropped under therapy with HES 70/0.5 from 2.5 to 1.1.

For a detailed discussion of the results refer to the original articles (Haaß et al. 1991, Treib et al. 1995–1997.

Discussion

For volume therapy, a variety of artificial colloidal plasma substitutes is available, which have in part significantly different, substance-specific properties. Studies regarding these substances are often limited to a one-time infusion of 500 to 1000 ml and are of limited value for a long-term volume therapy. Important criteria for the choice of a volume substitute are hemodynamic and rheological effectiveness and therapeutic safety.

Hemodynamic and Rheological Properties

The hemodynamic effect of a plasma substitute depends mostly on the *volume effect*. For the volume effect, the oncotic properties are more important than the concentration. Hyperoncotic solutions have plasma-expanding effects, because they bind additional volume intravascularly.

After a one-time infusion this volume-binding effect is approximately 100% for 10% Dextran 40 and HES 200/0.62, for 10% HES 200/0.5 it is approximately 50% (Köhler et al. 1982). According to the studies by Messmer and Jesch (1978) low molecular weight HES have no plasma-expanding effects.

Exsiccated patients in particular should receive sufficient amounts of electrolyte solution in addition to hyperoncotic plasma substitutes, to avoid the risk of increasing plasma viscosity (Haaß et al. 1989). The interstitial fluid deficit present in exsiccosis can be worsened through the infusion of plasma substitutes, because hyperoncotic solutions draw fluid from the interstitial space into the intravascular space. From a rheological perspective, electrolyte solution is not always necessary under therapy with a 6% solution, which has a weaker plasma-expanding effect.

The volume effect of such a solution is correspondingly lower. The hemodynamic effect depends on volume binding and plasma half-life and can be gauged by the hematocrit.

HES 200/0.62 has the strongest and longest-lasting volume effect (Fig. 28). One has to consider however that contrary to the other substances only 500 ml instead of 1000 ml were infused of the 10% solution in the first 4 days after the loading dose. The volume effect of the 0.5 substituted medium molecular weight HES solution is

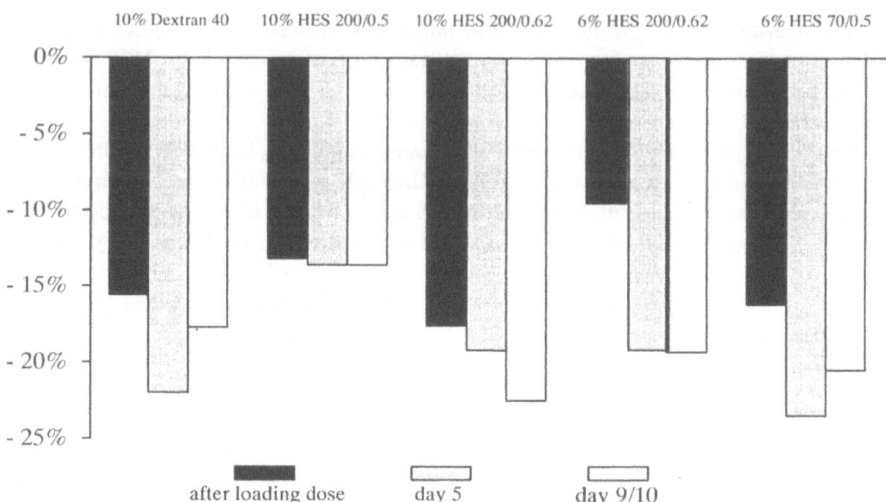

Fig. 28. Per cent change in hematocrit after long-term infusion of 10% HES 200/0.5, 10% Dextran 40, 10% HES 200/0.62 and 6% HES 70/0.5 (modified from Treib et al. 1997)

lowest overall, but the obtained lowering in hematocrit is sufficient for a rheologic therapy. The effect of 10% Dextran 40 lies between the two other solutions, yet one has to take into account that the volume effect of Dextran and more highly substituted HES lasts longer, because of the accumulation of larger molecules. The volume effect of low molecular weight HES is surprisingly high, because only a 6% solution was infused. But the volume effect depends less on the size of the molecules than on the number of oncotically active molecules. Immediately after the loading dose, hematocrit increased rapidly and dropped only after further high-dose therapy. A lasting hemodynamic effect can be achieved with this starch only through continuous infusion.

To judge the *rheological effectiveness*, one has to differentiate between the effect on micro- and macrocirculation. For the macrocirculation, the hematocrit and the full blood viscosity, which depends on the hematocrit, are of decisive importance. For the microcirculation on the other hand, the hematocrit, which is physiologically lower, is of lesser importance (Koscielny et al. 1991, Lin et al. 1995). Under impaired flow conditions, as they exist in the ischemic penumbra, erythrocyte aggregation and *plasma viscosity* are less relevant because of reduced perfusion pressure and frictional forces (Schmid-Schönbein 1982, Olsen et al. 1983). Due to the Fahraeus-Lindqvist effect, the effective viscosity of blood in the capillaries approaches the viscosity of plasma (Witzleb 1985). Plasma viscosity depends strongly on macromolecules in the plasma, such as fibrinogen. Large molecules increase erythrocyte aggregation when they bridge the physiological distance of approximately 30 nm between the erythrocytes (Chien et al. 1973 and 1981).

The importance of rheological factors for cerebral perfusion disorders is not widely known (Gaehtgens and Marx 1986). In patients with subcortical arteriosclerotic encephalopathy Ringelstein et al. (1988) were able to demonstrate the clinical relevance of fibrinogen concentration and plasma viscosity. By reducing the fibrinogen concentration from 326 mg/dl to 152 mg/dl, plasma viscosity decreased from 1.38 to 1.31 mPas. This led to a normalization of the cerebral perfusion reserve and an improvement of microcirculation, manifested by a 30% faster arterio-venous passage time in the retina. An acute improvement of cerebral competence or a long-lasting decline in the number of lacunar re-infarctions was not observed, so that the therapeutic effect of a fibrinogen and plasma-viscosity-lowering therapy was questioned.

The infusion of Dextran 40 and more highly substituted starch resulted in a pronounced increase of plasma viscosity during the therapy (Fig. 29). This increase paralleled *serum concentration* and depended on the concentration of the infusion solution and infusion velocity. Despite comparable serum concentrations (up to 20 mg/ml), HES 200/0.62 led to a smaller increase in plasma viscosity, because from a rheological perspective, the more spherically shaped HES molecules are more favorable than the chain-like configuration of Dextrans (Koscielny et al. 1991 and 1992). HES 200/0.5 and low molecular weight HES lower plasma viscosity, if suffdcent amounts of crystalloid fluids are infused.

Dextrans and HES also differ significantly in their effect on erythrocyte aggregation. Erythrocyte aggregation is caused by reversible bridge-binding between erythrocytes which can approach each other only up to a distance of 30 nm, because of repulsive Coloumb forces. Erythrocytes can only attach to each other when larger molecules, such as fibrinogen, form "bridges" between the erythrocyte membranes (Chien and Jan 1973 and 1981). Smaller molecules on the other hand can crowd out the aggregation-supporting macromolecules and therefore have an aggregation-inhibiting effect.

While Dextran, due to its chain-like shape can increase erythrocyte aggregation already at molecule sizes above 60,000 D, starch with its more spherical shape exerts

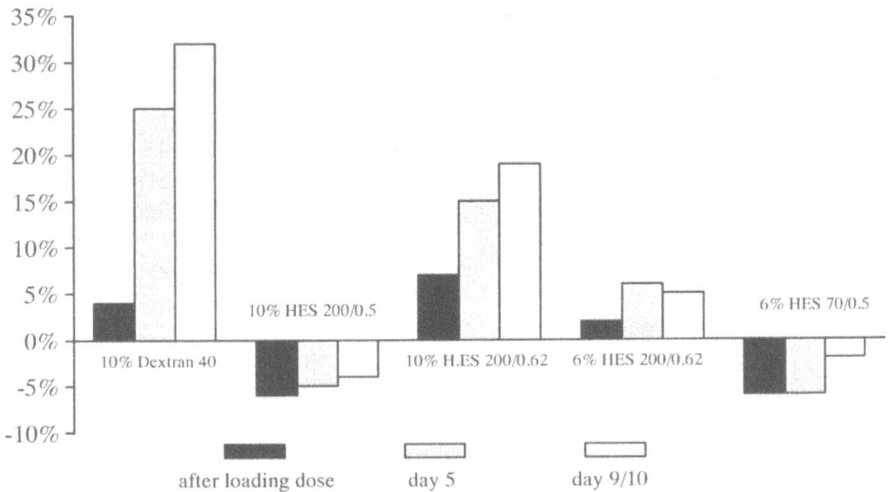

Fig. 29. Per cent change in plasma viscosity after long-term infusion of 10% HES 200/0.5, 10% Dextran 40, 10% HES 200/0.62 and 6% HES 70/0.5

this effect only at molecule sizes of several hundred thousand Dalton (Treib et al. 1991). Dextran, which causes a decrease in erythrocyte aggregation after a single infusion, leads to a steady increase in aggregation after repeated infusion over several days. HES on the other hand improves this parameter after repeated infusion. Only after infusion of high doses of the more highly substituted HES, aggregation increases slightly.

One explanation for this differing behaviour can be found in the examination of the in-vivo molecular weight. In a single, short infusion of Dextran, the smaller molecules, which lower the tendency to aggregate, dominate. After repeated, slow infusion, larger molecules that are difficult to eliminate accumulate, leading to an increase in erythrocyte aggregation.

Starch molecules, on the other hand, are metabolized in-vivo and the resulting small molecules lower erythrocyte aggregation. Only a loading dose of 10% HES 200/0.62 leads through the massive presence of large molecules to an increase in aggregation. With continuing therapy, however, the large molecules are broken down enzymatically and smaller, aggregation-inhibiting molecules dominate. Through a loading dose of low molecular weight HES many small molecules appear in the blood, slowing aggregation. After long-term infusion therapy, smaller molecules are eliminated and aggregation increases again. HES 200/0.5 has the strongest aggregation-lowering effect, which reaches its maximum effect at the end of therapy.

The differing rheological properties of the studied substances are due to their differing *molecular weight distribution*. After infusing Dextran 40, with an in-vitro molecular weight of 52,000 D, larger molecules cumulate in-vivo and Mw reaches twice the initial value. HES, on the other hand, is metabolized rapidly in-vivo through alpha-amylases.

The in-vitro Mw of the HES 200/0.5 infusion solution is 200,000 D. In-vivo, this substance is broken down quickly, so that small HES molecules with an average Mw of 84,000 D are responsible for the biological effects. Highly substituted HES 200/0.62 is broken down slowly, the average Mw in-vivo is much higher at 120,000 D. Because elimination is more difficult, macromolecules accumulate, raising serum concentration up 20 mg/ml. Low molecular weight HES hardly changes its initial Mw (60,000 D) and has favorable rheologic properties, similar to HES 200/0.5. Both substances do not lead to an increase in serum concentration.

Boldt et al. (1994) observed a pronounced increase in plasma viscosity after a hemodilution therapy with HES 450/0.7. Because of the high initial Mw and the high degree of substitution, this starch solution has a high in-vivo Mw, which explains the increase in plasma viscosity.

Platelet Count and Function

None of the solutions studied caused a decrease in platelet count that went beyond the dilution effect. After an initial dilution-induced decrease in platelet count, the number of platelets increased during the therapy, possibly the result of a reactive release of platelets. For the starch solutions, platelet volume was also measured. All the HES solutions caused a small, yet significant decrease in platelet volume.

The decline in platelet volume seems to be a dose-dependent effect, because 10% HES 200/0.62 led to a 40% larger drop in platelet volume than 6% HES 200/0.62. The more highly substituted HES 200/0.62 caused a larger decrease in platelet volume than HES 200/0.5 and HES 70/0.5. Our analysis of the molecular weight distribution showed that the decline in platelet volume was more pronounced, if the in-vivo Mw of the HES was higher (Treib et al. 1996).

The decline in platelet volume, is most likely the result of a shrinkage of the platelets, due to increased colloid-osmotic pressure. This hypothesis is supported by the fact that platelet count at the maximum value and distribution width of the platelets remained constant (Treib et al. 1996). An increased break-down or phagocytosis of platelets after attaching to HES can also not be excluded, because platelets are a part of the unspecific immune defenses of the body and play an important role in the phagocytosis and elimination of foreign particles (Kemona et al. 1986). It is also possible that platelet microaggregates are dissolved through hemodynamic and rheological effects and augmented shear stress phenomena. The dissolution of these reversible platelet aggregates would increase the number of platelets counted and seemingly lower the mean platelet volume, explaining the increasing platelet count and decreasing platelet volume.

The diagnostic importance of decreasing platelet volume is unclear (Levin and Bessman 1983, Bessman et al. 1985, Erne et al. 1988, Kristensen et al. 1988, Threatte 1993). Several studies showed that a positive correlation exists between platelet volume, -function and bleeding time (Karpatkin 1978, Eldor et al. 1982, Thompson et al. 1982, Kristensen et al. 1988). Therefore, one can suspect that platelet function is impaired during a volume therapy with HES. The significant decline of platelet volume observed in this study seems to have only a small effect on platelet volume, because platelet aggregation is slightly impaired only through the infusion of 10% HES 200/0.62.

Dextran solutions on the other hand impair platelet aggregation more than starches (Harke et al. 1976 and 1980, Popov-Cenic 1977, Haaß et al. 1986). They are suited less for the acute therapy of a stroke, because intracerebral hemorrhage has to be excluded with cranial CT before therapy can be initiated (Hartmann 1987). When infusing starches, a desired inhibition of platelet aggregation can be achieved with acetyl salicylic acid after exclusion of an intracerebral hemorrhage (Treib and Haaß 1999).

Plasmatic Coagulation System

The severe hemorrhagic complications observed after repeated infusion of highly subsituted, high molecular weight HES 480/0.7 (hetastarch) underline the clinical relevance of coagulation disorders induced through plasma substitutes (Symington 1986, Damon et al. 1987, Bianchine 1987, Cully et al. 1987, Sanfelippo et al. 1988, Lockwood et al. 1988, Abramson 1988, Trumble et al. 1995).

In our studies the reduction of *thromboplastin time (quick)* was most pronounced for Dextran (23%), followed by HES 200/0.62 (-20%). After infusion of HES 200/0.5 or low molecular weight HES, no relevant changes in thromboplastin time were observed.

Depending on the substance used, the dose and duration of therapy, *PTT* is affected differently. Infusion of low molecular weight HES and HES 200/0.5 resulted in

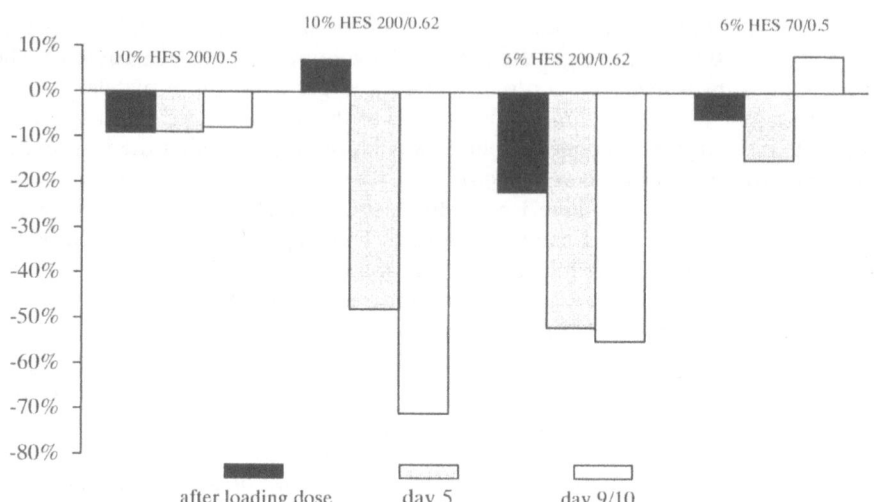

Fig. 30. Per cent change in factor VIII:C after long-term infusion of 10% HES 200/0.5, 10% Dextran 40, 10% HES 200/0.62 and 6% HES 70/0.5 (modified from Treib et al. 1997)

no notable effect on PTT beyond the dilution effect. Infusion of Dextran 40 increased PTT by 24%, infusion of 10% HES 200/0.62 by 43%.

The prolonged PTT time indicates an impairment of the intrinsic system of coagulation, mostly due to an impairment of factor VIII/vWF complex (Fig. 30). The importance of the von Willebrand factor lies in the attachment of platelets to the damaged vascular endothelium. A shortage of von Willebrand factor rarely leads to spontaneous bleeding, but afterbleedings even after minor injury can be considerably prolonged. Half of the patients with Ristocetin cofactor values of 40–45% have a history of bleeding (Krentzlin et al. 1985). HES 200/0.5 and HES 70/0.5 hardly affect factor VIII:C, von Willebrand factor antigen and Ristocetin co-factor. However, after repeated infusion of HES 200/0.62 factor VIII/vWF complex dropped regularly below the hemostasiological limit of 30%. Yet, none of our patients suffered from clinically relevant hemorrhagic complications that needed treatment. Only one patient had spontaneous gum bleeding.

The lowering of factor VIII:C in von Willebrand syndrome is probably a secondary consequence of the lowering in vWF, because vWF has a stabilizing function as a carrier protein for factor VIII:C (Budde et al. 1986).

How HES affects factor VIII/vWF complex is still largely unknown. After the addition of HES to human serum in in-vitro studies, Batlle et al. (1985) and Stump et al. (1985) did not observe a decrease in factor VIII/vWF complex that went beyond the dilution effect. The authors therefore suspected the occurrence of an in-vivo precipitation or an inhibition of synthesis or release. Because patients with monoclonal gammopathy suffer from an acquired von Willebrand syndrome (Siostrzonek et al. 1985, Ruggeri 1994, Arkel et al. 1994), an accelerated elimination of factor VIII/vWF complex after attachment of HES molecules is another possible explanation. The finding of a factor VIII-IgG-paraprotein complex by Siostrzonek et al. (1985) supports this hypothesis. The authors explained the low factor VIII levels and the rapid drop after administration of cryoprecipitate or desamino-D-arginine vasopressin (DDAVP) with an accelerated elimination of the complex. The successful treatment of an acquired von Willebrand syndrome with immuno globulins lends further credence to the view of an immune-system modulated mechanism (Arkel et al. 1994).

In our study, we were able to show for the first time through vWF multimeric analysis that all multimer components are reduced to the same extent by the infusion therapy. The coagulation disorder caused by HES is therefore a purely quantitative defect, corresponding to type I von Willebrand syndrome (Zimmermann and Ruggeri 1983, Ruggeri 1994, Treib et al. 1996). Because the coagulation disorder caused by HES was classified for the first time, it was possible to consider possible therapies, since particularly type I von Willebrand syndrome can be treated with the vasopressin derivative DDAVP (Holmberg and Nilsson 1985).

The coagulation disorder observed under therapy with highly substituted starch could be of therapeutic interest, because the use of this starch could be therapeutically useful in patients with an increased risk of thrombosis or reinfarction.

Our studies showed differing effects of the individual starches on coagulation parameters. According to our studies, the drop in factor VIII/vWF complex correlates with the dose, the initial molecular weight, the share of C2-hydroxyethylated starch molecules and particularly the molar substitution ratio of the starch. This is the case because the larger molecules that are difficult to eliminate are responsible for the coagulation disorder. Therefore, hemorrhagic complications can be avoided through the choice of a suitable starch with a low in-vivo Mw (Treib et al. 1995–1999).

A shortening of *thrombin time* and a lowering of *fibrinogen concentration* after a single infusion of Dextran or HES has been described repeatedly in the literature (Peter et al. 1975, Vinazzer and Bergmann 1975, Popov-Cenic et al. 1977, Költringer et al. 1989). These effects are probably due to accelerated polymerization of fibrin. For hemostasis, they are of secondary importance. The largest decrease can be observed for Dextran and highly substituted HES, whereas HES 200/0.5 and low molecular weight HES lead to no relevant changes in thrombin time and fibrinogen concentration.

Factors XI and XII are reduced through highly substituted starch by approximately one-half. This indicates that the impairment of the intrinsic system is not limited to factor VIII/vWF complex. Significant drops of factor XI and XII can be avoided through the use of low molecular weight HES 70/0.5 or HES 200/0.5.

In addition, a small, clinically not relevant reduction in *factor II and X* was observed. *Factors V, VII and IX* were not affected beyond the dilution effect.

Neither the concentration or the activity of *C1-inactivator*, a central inhibitor of coagulation factor XI and XII showed significant changes during the therapy. The average drop in activity of factor XI and XII can therefore not be explained through a change in C1-inhibitor (Barthels and Poliwoda 1987).

Thrombin is a key enzyme for the formation of fibrin from fibrinogen, antithrombin III is its physiological inhibitor. An increased concentration of *thrombin/antithrombin III (TAT) complex* shows an intravascular activation of coagulation and an increased tendeny for thrombosis (Blanke et al. 1987). However, we did not observe any significant changes in the TAT III complex under a volume therapy with HES.

Fibronectin and ReticuloEndothelial System (RES)

Fibronectin (Fn) is important for the non-immune-specific "clearing" function of the RES, an important defense mechanism of the body. Fn acts as opsonin, it has binding sites for phagocytosing RES cells as well as for different target molecules such as collagen, gelatin, fibrinogen, fibrin and bacteria (Doran 1983, Mork and Hancock 1993, Xie et al. 1993, Ratliff et al. 1993).

In animal experiments, the RES can be blocked through repeated administration of gelatin particles (Saba and Cho 1969). According to studies by Saba, inhibition of RES is associated with a reduction in Fn. In animal experiments, the elimination acitivity of RES increased again after the administration of Fn (Saba and Cho 1979). However, more recent studies showed only a limited correlation between RES function and Fn plasma concentration (Lunsgaard-Hansen et al. 1986, Powell and Doran 1991).

From a pathophysiological perspective, an impairment of Fn and the RES through colloidal plasma substitutes seems plausible. In particular plasma substitutes with a high initial molecular weight that are slowly eliminated via the kidneys are probably eliminated to a considerable extent via the RES.

Therapy-resistent pruritus, the most frequent side effect after repeated infusion of HES is also associated with the RES (Kiesewetter et al. 1992). The dose-dependency and the long latency until the occurrence of the complaint suggest that they are the consequence of extravascular HES deposits. This is supported by the observation that human monocytes and keratinocytes can ingest and store HES (Szepfalusi et al. 1993). Thompson et al. (1979) observed in animal studies that after one day 30–43% of the infused HES was located in the extravascular space. In dogs, temporary storage in liver, spleen, kidneys and lymph nodes was observed. HES granula were found in the interstitial space, liver parenchyma cells, renal tubule cells and in phagocytes of the liver, spleen and lymph nodes.

The mechanism of HES uptake in the extravascular space is unclear. The observed drop in fibronectin suggests that Fn acts as an opsonin. Possibly, Fn plays a central role in the coagulation disorders observed under therapy with HES, because Fn has a special affinity to vWF, fibrinogen and platelets (Pearlstein et al. 1980, Giddings 1987, Connellan et al. 1991, Burnouf-Radosevich and Burnouf 1992, Bos et al. 1993, Difazio et al. 1994).

In our studies, we showed that the in-vivo Mw of HES is of decisive importance for the extent of the coagulation disorders observed during therapy with HES. The decline in Fn parallels the decline of factor VIII/vWF. Because of the high affinity of Fn to von Willebrand factor, a comparable elimination mechanism can be suspected (Pearlstein et al. 1980, Burnouf-Radosevich and Burnouf 1992, Bos et al. 1993, Difazio et al. 1994).

Further studies are necessary to examine the possible clinical relevance of the observed decrease in Fn, besides the impairment of the RES and coagulation. A 10-day volume therapy with HES 200/0.5 (1) lead to a significant increase of neutrophilic granulocytes, which also have a Fn receptor at the cell surface (Lukowsky et al. 1986, Yang et al. 1994). Since Fn also plays an important role in embryogenesis, wound healing and unspecific immune defense, effects on these systems are also possible.

It is unknown which Fn concentration is necessary for normal functioning of the RES. Patients with a 50% lower Fn concentration have a higher mortality (Mosher and Furcht 1981). Non-surviving intensive care patients have lower concentrations than surviving patients, but this could also be due to generally low plasma proteins. One study of patients with severe abdominal infections reported a statistically not significant lowering of mortality after administration of Fn (Lundsgaard et al. 1986). Later studies could not prove the efficacy of a Fn therapy for trauma and sepsis patients (Powell and Duran 1991).

The decrease in Fn after several HES infusions measured in our study does not necessarily mean the RES depression is clinically relevant. Several studies yielded contradictory results and showed no clear RES depression after infusion of colloids. After administration of HES, oxypolygelatin and human albumin, Lenz et al. (1986) did not observe an impairment of RES phagocytosis activity in healthy humans, but an increase of Fn. Shatney and Chaudry (1984) also did not observe RES depression after administration of HES. Schildt et al. (1975) on the other hand found a reduction in phagocytosis activity in mice with burn injuries after administration of colloids.

Earlier studies showed no decrease in plasma fibronectin after infusion of colloids that went beyond the dilution effect (Khosropour et al. 1984, Brodin et al. 1984, Lackner et al. 1985). Contrary to our study, the effect on Fn was only measured after a single infusion and not during the course of a hemodilution therapy over several days. Analysis of our data shows that Fn drops on day 1 within the range of the dilution effect. While hematocrit remains approximately constant, Fn decreases continuously until the last day of infusions. In the group with the high-dose 10% HES 200/0.62 solution, Fn continues to drop after the end of infusion therapy. Therefore, Fn decrease beyond the dilution effect occurs only after repeated infusion of starch. This indicates that Fn reservoirs are only exhausted after repeated administration of plasma substitutes.

Highly substituted, high molecular weight HES preparations with a high intravascular molecular weight should therefore be used with caution in patients suffering from coagulation disorders, organ failure, sepsis, extensive burns and wounds. Large doses and long therapies should be avoided. In these cases, low and medium molecular weight starch with a low degree of substitution should be preferred. Besides a more favorable effect on rheological and hemostasiological parameters they probably affect Fn less (Treib et al. 1996 and 1998).

Amylases, Lipases, and Blood Count

During an infusion therapy for 9 to 10 days with HES 200/0.62, *serum amylases* increased more than five-fold. After the end of therapy, this increase is only slowly reversible, as can be seen from the concentration on day 9 to 13. The increase of amylases after infusion of HES solution has been described repeatedly (Misher 1980, Köhler et al. 1982, Költringer et al. 1989). This hyperamylasemia is not clinically relevant, because the pancreas or other organ systems are not affected. This is confirmed by the normal *lipase activity*. One has to consider that during therapy and a few days afterwards, the serum amylases cannot be used diagnostically. The examination of the *blood count* was normal and showed only dilution effects, except for a small increase in neutrophilic granulocytes.

HES Substitution Pattern

We studied the effects of different substitution patterns on rheology and coagulation system with two starches that differed in their C_2/C_6 ratio and were identical in concentration, initial molecular weight molar substitution ratio (Treib et al. 1995). The C_2/C_6 ratio of 10% HES 200/0.5 (1) was 13.4, for HES 200/0.5 (2) it was 5.7.

Yoshida et al. (1984) showed in animal experiments that 2-hydroxyethylated starch is metabolized more slowly. Our studies confirmed this. Hematocrit was lowered in both groups through the loading dose equally by 18%. During the further therapy however, HES (1) with the lower elimination rate had a longer-lasting volume effect and the maximum decrease in hematocrit was significantly larger than in the other group (30.5% vs. 23.5%). Erythrocyte aggregation was affected favorably by both substances. The effect was more pronounced for HES (1) at 41% reduction. The continuous increase in plasma viscosity measured for HES (1) was higher than for HES (2).

The starch with the higher C_2/C_6 ratio has more unfavorable effects on the coagulation system. PTT increase was more pronounced (30%) for HES (1) than for HES (2) (13%). Factor VIII:C was also more reduced by HES (1) than HES (2) (-64% vs. 19%, respectively). The longer-lasting volume effect, the larger increase in plasma viscosity and the greater impairment of the coagulation system caused by HES (1) are due to an accumulation of large molecules that are difficult to eliminate. This is confirmed by the serum concentrations and the distribution of the molecular weight. The higher share of C_2-hydroxyethylated starch that is difficult to break down resulted in a continous increase of serum concentration up to 15 mg/ml through the infusion of HES 200/0.5 (1). Maximum serum concentration in group 2 was 10 mg/ml. The analysis of molecular weight distribution showed that the Mw of HES (1) immediately after the loading dose was higher than for HES (2) (144,000 vs. 118,000 D, respectively). At the end of therapy, the values were 95,000 D for group 1 and 84,000 D for group 2.

Because of their different substitution patterns, the three HES solution studied, all labeled 10% HES 200/0.5 differ significantly in their hemostasiological and rheological properties. HES 200/0.5 has the smallest volume effect, but at the same time this preparation has the most favorable rheological properties and does not impair the coagulation system. HES 200/0.5 (1), with the higher C_2/C_6 ratio is metabolized slowly and has very similar characteristics to HES 200/0.62. HES 200/0.5 (2) occupies a middle position among the three starches, regarding volume effect and hemostasiological and rheologial properties (Haaß et al. 1991, Treib et al. 1996, Treib et al. 1998).

Oxygen Carrying Plasma Substitutes for the Volume Therapy of the Future

For the volume therapy of brain stroke, all studied plasma substitutes have the disadvantage that although they increase cerebral blood flow through a reduction in viscosity, at the same time they reduce the oxygen-carrying capacity of the blood through dilution (Leonov et al. 1992). In the future, this disadvantage can maybe be compensated for through the use of oxygen-binding plasma substitutes. In an animal stroke model, Kline et al. (1991) found evidence for the superiority of perflurocarbon emulsions in a stroke model. After interrupting the middle cerebral artery and subsequent isovolemic hemodilution with a perfluorcarbon emulsion or Dextran 40, they observed in perfluorcarbon-treated cats a significantly (p<0.05) smaller ischemic brain edema than in the Dextran group. There was no significant difference in hemodynamic and rheological parameters. Although the second generation of perflurocarbons, so-called perflurocytylbromides (PFOB) and hemoglobin solutions are currently tested clinically, it will certainly take several more years until these promising substances can be used routinely (Keipert 1995, Lee et al. 1995, Spence 1995, Spahn 1998). Another interesting field of study would be the efficacy of gelatin solutions for hemodynamically and rheologically oriented volume therapy.

Evaluation of the Plasma Substitutes

Dextran 40 as well as high- and medium molecular weight *HES 450/0.7 and HES 200/ 0.62*, both of which are difficult to break down, have a longer-lasting volume effect. However, they cannot be recommended for a volume therapy over several days, because their difficult elimination leads to an accumulation of large molecules. These macromolecues affect the coagulation system via a decrease in factor VIII/vWF complex, resulting in increased hemorrhagic risk, increased plasma viscosity and impaired erythrocyte aggregation. Dextran increases the risk of bleeding through an inhibition of platelet aggregation and has the added disadvantage of a higher incidence of anaphylactoid reactions (Messmer and Jesch 1978, Sommermeyer et al. 1987, Lang 1992).

Easily degradable, medium molecular weight *HES 200/0.5* has a medium volume effect and duration. With a suitable substitution pattern, the starch molecules are broken down rapidly in-vivo to rheologically favorable molecule sizes. During a long-term therapy, no relevant cumulation or increase in hemorrhages occurs. This plasma substitute can therefore be recommended for volume therapy.

Low molecular weight starch (HES 70/0.5) has very favorable rheological and hemostasiological properties. Its volume effect, however is shorter. Due to the short

Table 3. Influence of Dextran 40, HES 200/0.5, HES 200/0.62 and HES 70/0.5 on hemostasis and hemorrheology

	Dextran 40	HES 200/0.5	HES 200/0.62	HES 70/0.5
Molecular weight (MW)				
In vitro	52000	200000	270000	60000
In vivo	102000	84000	120000	57000
Hematocrit	↓↓	↓	↓↓	↓
Eryaggregation	↑↑	↓	↑↓	↓
Plasma viscosity	↑↑	↓	↑	↓
PTT	↑	o	↑↑	o
Factor VIII/vWF	↓	o	↓↓	o

volume effect, this substance should be infused more frequently or continuously. This substance should be used when the rheological aspect of the volume therapy is more important than the hemodynamic effect (Table 3).

References

Abramson N: Plasma Expanders and Bleeding. Ann Intern Med 108, 307, 1988
Appel PL, Kram HB, MacKabee J, Fleming AW, Shoemaker WC: Comparison of measurements of cardiac output by bioimpedance and thermodilution in severely ill surgical patients. Crit Care Med 14, 933–935, 1986
Appel PL, Shoemaker WC: Fluid therapy in adult respiratory failure. Crit Care Med 9, 862, 1981
Arkel YS, Lynch J, Kamiyama M: Treatment of acquired von Willebrand syndrome with intravenous immunoglobulin. Thromb Haemost 72, 643–51, 1994
Baron J-F, Treib J (eds.) Volume Replacement. Springer, Berlin-Heidelberg-New York, 1–143, 1998
Barthels M, Poliwoda H (Hrsg) Gerinnungsanalysen. Thieme, Stuttgart, 1987
Batlle J, Del Rio F, Fernandez M F, Martin R, Borrasca A: Effect of dextran on factor VIII / von Willebrand factor structur and function. Thromb Haemost 54, 697–699, 1985
Beards SC, Watt T, Edwards JD, Nightingale P, Farragher B: Comparison of the hemodynamic and oxygen transport responses to modified fluid gelatin and hetastarch in critically ill patients: A prospective, randomized trial. Crit Care Med 22, 600–605, 1994
Bessman JD, Gilmer PR, Gardner FH: Use of mean platelet volume improves detection of platelet disorders. Blood cells 11, 127–135, 1985
Bianchine JR: To the editor. N Engl J Med 317, 965, 1987
Biggs R, Mac Farlane RG: Human blood coagulation and its disorders. Blachwell Scientific Publications, Oxford 1962
Blanke H, Praetorius G, Leschke M, Seitz R, Egbring R, Strauer BE: Die Bedeutung des Thrombin-Antithrombin III-Komplexes in der Diagnostik der Lungenembolie und der tiefen Venenthrombose. Klin Wschr 65, 757–763, 1987
Boldt J, Knothe C, Zickmann B, Ballesteros M, Zeiler D, Dapper F, Hempelmann G: Kardiorespiratorische und mikrozirkulatorische Effekte nach Volumenersatz mit einer neuen Hydroxyethylstärke-Präparation. Anaesthesist 41, 316–323, 1992
Boldt J, Zickmann B, Rapin J, Hammermann H, Dapper F, Hempelmann G: Influence of volume replacement with different HES-solutions on microcirculatory blood flow in cardiac surgery. Acta Anaesthesiol Scand 38, 432–438, 1994
Bos AN, Post MJ, de Groot PG, Sixma JJ, Borst C: Both increased and decreased platelet adhesion to thermal injured subendothelium is caused by denaturation of von Willebrand factor. Circulation 88, 1196–1204, 1993
Böttcher, Brockhaus, Hellstern, Klose, Rasche, Schimpf, Scharrer, Schramm, Wenzel: Die PTT verschiedener Hersteller als Suchtest von Faktor VIII-Mangelzuständen. in: Landbeck G, Marx R, Stolte HP (Hrsg) 10. Hämophilie-Symposion Hamburg, Pharmazeutische Verlagsgesellschaft, München, 1979
Bredin K, Grun H, Krzywanek HJ, Schremmer WP: Zur Messung der "spontanen" Thrombozyten aggregation. Plättchenaggregationstest III. Methodik. Klin Wschr 53, 81–89, 1975
Brodin B, Hesselvik F, von Schenk H: Decrease of plasma fibronectin concentration following infusion of a gelatin-based plasma substitute in man. Scand J clin Lab Invest 44, 529–533, 1984
Bsteh M, Tews G, John D: Hämodilution bei der Behandlung der intrauterinen Dystrophie. Geburtsh Frauenheilk 55, 83–86, 1995
Budde U, Steinberg A: Analyse der Multimere und Polypeptide des von Willebrand-Faktors. In: Landbeck G (Hrsg) 16. Hämophilie Symposion, Hamburg. Springer, Berlin Heidelberg New York, 179–183, 1985
Burnouf-Radosevich M, Burnouf T: Chromatographic preparation of therapeutic highly purified von Willebrand factor concentrate from human cryoprecipitate. Vox Sang 62, 1–11, 1992
Camu F, Ivens D, Christiaens F: Human albumine and colloid fluid replacement: their use in general surgery. Acta Anaesthesiol Belg 46, 3–18, 1995

Chien S, Jan KM: Ultrastructural basis of the mechanism of rouleaux formation. Mikrovask Res 5, 155–166, 1973

Chien S: Determinats of blood viscosity and red cell deformability. J Clin Lab Invest 40, 7–12, 1981

Clauss, Ebner: Statistik für Soziologen, Pädagogen, Psychologen und Mediziner. Harri Deutsch, Thun 1985

Connellan JM, Deacon S, Thurlow PJ: Changes in platelet function and reactivity induced by quinine in relation to quinine (drug) induced immune thrombocytopenia. Thrombos Res 61, 501–514, 1991

Cully MD, Larson CP, Silverberg GD: Hetastarch coagulopathy in a neurosurgical patient. Anaesthesiology 66, 707–708, 1987

Damon L, Adams M, Stricker RB, Ries C: Intracranial bleeding during treatment with hydroxyethyl starch. N Engl J Med 317, 964–965, 1987

DiFazio LT, Stratoulias C, Greco RS, Haimovich B: Multiple platelet surface receptors mediate platelet adhesion to surfaces coated with plasma proteins. J Surg Res 57, 133–137, 1994

Doran JE: A critical assessment of fibronectin's opsonic role for bacteria and microaggregates. Vox Sang 45, 337–348, 1983

Ehrly AM, Landgraf H, Saeger-Lorenz K, Hasse S: Verbesserung der Fließeigenschaften nach Infusion von niedermolekularer Hydroxyäthylstärke (Expafusin) bei gesunden Probanden. Infusionstherapie 6, 331–336, 1979

Ehrly AM, Seebens H, Saeger-Lorenz K: Einfluß einer 10%igen und 6%igen Hydroxyäthylstärkelösung (MG 200000/0,62) im Vergleich mit einer 10%igen Dextranlösung (MG 40000) auf die Fließeigenschaften des Blutes und den Gewebesauerstoffdruck von Patienten mit Claudicatio intermittens. Infusionstherapie 15, 181–187, 1988

Eigner W-D: Hydroxyethylstärke, Molmassenbestimmung von Hydroxyethylstärke in Elektrolytlösung nach Temperaturbelastung. Krankenhauspharmazie 9, 20–22, 1988

Eldor A, Avitzour M, Or R, Hanna R, Penchas S: Prediction of haemorrhagic diathesis in thrombocytopenia by mean platelet volume. Brit Med J 285, 397–400, 1982

Erne P, Wardle J, Sanders K, Lewis SM, Maseri A: Mean platelet volume and size distribution and their sensitivity to agonists in patients with coronary artery disease and congestive heart failure. Thromb Haemost 59, 259–263, 1988

Förster H, Wicarkzyk C, Dudziak R: Bestimmung der Plasmaelimination von Hydroxyäthylstärke und von Dextran mittels verbesserter analytischer Methodik. Infusionstherapie 2, 88–94, 1981

Funk W, Baldinger V: Microcirculatory perfusion during volume therapy. A comperative study using crystalloid or colloid in awake animals. Anesthesilogy 82, 975–982, 1995

Gaehtgens P, Marx P: Hemorheological aspects of the pathophysiology of cerebral ischemia. J Cereb Blood Flow Metab 7, 259–265, 1987

Giddings JC: Localisation and synthesis of fibronectin. In: Bloom AL and Thomas DP (eds): Haemostasis and thrombosis, Churchill Livingstone, Edinburgh London Melbourne New York, 313–315, 1987

Gottstein U, Held K: Effekt der Hämodilution nach intravenöser Infusion von niedermolekularen Dextranen auf die Hirnzirkulation des Menschen. Dtsch Med Wschr 11, 522–526, 1969

Grauer MT, Treib J: The effect of hydroxyethyl starch on coagulation is difficult to assess in vitro. British Journal of Anaesthesia 80, 125–126, 1998

Haaß A, Kroemer H, Jäger H, Oest A, Heinrich B: Hemodilution therapie in cerebral ischemia, different dose- and timedependent hemorheological effects of plasma expanders. In: Kriegelstein J (ed): Pharmacology of cerebral ischemia. Elsevier, Amsterdam, 1986

Haaß A, Kroemer H, Jäger H, Müller K, Decker I, Wagner EM, Schimrigk K: Dextran 40 oder HES 200/0,5 ? Hämorheologie der Langzeitbehandlung beim ischämischen zerebralen Insult. Dtsch Med Wschr 111, 1681–1686, 1986

Haaß A, Kroemer H, Jäger H, Oest A, Schimrigk K: Similar and opposite hemorheological effects of dextran 40 and hydroxyethyl starch in hemodilution therapie for stroke. In: Hartmann A and Kuschinsky W (eds.): Cerebral ischemia and hemorheology. Springer, Berlin-Heidelberg, 1987

Haaß A: Hämodilution mit mittelmolekularer Stärke zur Therapie des ischämischen Insultes, der Subarachnoidalblutung und intrazerebralen Blutung, hämorheologische und gerinnungsphysiologische Probleme. In: Lawin P (Hrsg): Hydroxyäthylstärke, eine aktuelle Übersicht. Thieme, Stuttgart New York, 1989

Haaß A: Therapie des akuten ischämischen Insultes. Nervenheilkunde 8, 35–45, 1989

Haaß A: Hämorheologische Therapie, Stand und Perspektiven. Nervenarzt 60, 528–539, 1989

Haaß A: Hämodilutionstherapie beim ischämischen Hirninfarkt: Sinnvoll. Akt Neurol 16, 213–219, 1989
Haaß A, Stoll M, Treib J: Hämodilution bei cerebralen Durchblutungsstörungen. Indikation, Durchführung, medikamentöse Zusatzbehandlung und Alternativen. In: Koscielny J, Kiesewetter H, Jung F, Haaß A (Hrsg): Hämodilution, neue Aspekte in der Behandlung von Durchblutungsstörungen. Springer, Berlin-Heidelberg, 1991
Haaß A, Stoll M, Treib J, Krack P, Decker I, Hamann G, Kässer U: Hämorheologische und hämodynamische Befunde und ihre klinische Bedeutung für die Hämodilution. In: Landgraf H, Ehrly AM (Hrsg): Hämodilution bei akuter zerebraler Ischämie. Blackwell Wissenschaft, Berlin, 1992
Haaß A, Treib J, Stoll M: Hemorheological parameters of hydroxyethyl starch 200/0,62 as a basis for hemodilution. Clin Hemorheol 12, Supp. 1, 17–26, 1992
Hankeln K, Rädel C, Beez M, Laniewski P, Bohmert F: Comparison of hydroxyethyl starch and lactated Ringer's solution on hemodynamics and oxygen transport of critically ill patients in prospective crossover studies. Crit Care Med 17, 133–135, 1989
Hankeln K, Senker R, Beez M: Comparative study of the intraoperative efficacy of 5% human albumine and 10% hydroxyethyl starch (HES-steril) in terms of hemodynamics and oxygen transport in 40 patients. Infusionsther Transfusionsmed 17, 135–140, 1990
Hansen D, Hannemann L, Specht M, Schaffartzik W: Zerebraler Vasospasmus nach aneurysmatischer Subarachnoidalblutung. Therapeutischer Stellenwert von Kalzium-antagonisten, hypervolämischer Hämodilution und induzierter arterieller Hypertension. Anaesthesist 44, 219–229, 1995
Harke H, Thoenies R, Margraf I, Momsen W: Der Einfluß verschiedener Plasmaersatzmittel auf Gerinnungssystem und Thrombozytenfunktion während und nach operativen Eingriffen. Anaesthesist 25, 366–373, 1976
Harke H, Pieper C, Meredig J, Rahman S, Rüssler P: Rheologische und gerinnungsphysiologische Untersuchungen nach Infusion von HÄS 200/0,5 und Dextran 40. Anaesthesist 29, 71–77, 1980
Hartmann A: Die Hämodilution beim zerebralen Insult. Akt Neurol 14, 42–49, 1987
Heber H, Kolde HJ, Heimburger N, Svendsen G: New chromogenic substrate for C1-inhibitor functional activity assay. Thromb Haemost 50, 227, 1983
Holmberg L, Nilsson IM: Von Willebrand disease. Clin Haematol 14, 461–488, 1985
Jung F, Roggenkamp HG, Schneider R, Kiesewetter H: Das Kapillarschlauch-Plasmaviskosimeter, ein neues Meßgerät zur Quantifizierung der Blutplasmaviskosität. Biomed Technik 28, 249–252, 1983
Jung F, Waldhausen P, Spitzer S, Mrowietz C, Häuser B, Wenzel E: Hämorheologische, mikro- und makrozirkulatorische Effekte einer hypervolämischen Hämodilution mit mittelmolekularer Hydroxyäthylstärke (HES 200/0,62; 6%). Infusionstherapie 15, 266–271, 1988
Jung F, Koscielny J, Kolepke W, Scheffler P, Kiesewetter H, Wenzel E: Einfluß einer iso- bzw. hyper volämischen Hämodilution auf die Fließfähigkeit des Blutes, die Sauerstoff-transportkapazität in der Makro- und Mikrostrombahn sowie die Gewebesauerstoffversorgung von Haut- und Skelettmuskel. In: Lawin P (Hrsg): Hydroxyäthylstärke – eine aktuelle Übersicht. Thieme, Stuttgart New York, 1989
Karlson KE, Garzon AA, Shaftan GW, Chu C-J: Increased blood loss associated with administration of certain plasma expanders: Dextran 75, dextran 40 and hydroxyethyl starch. Surgery 62, 670–678, 1967
Karpatkin S: Heterogeneity of human platelets, correlation of platelet function with platelet volume. Blood 51, 307–316, 1978
Keipert PE: Use of Oxygent, a perflurochemical-based oxygen carrier as an alternative to intraoperative blood transfusion. Art Cells Blood Subs and Immob Biotech 23, 381–394, 1995
Kemona H, Andrzejewska A, Prokopowicz J, Nowak H, Mantur M: Phagocytic activity of human blood platelets examined by electron microscopy. Folia Haematol 113, 696–702, 1986
Khosropour R, Graninger W, Lackner F: Der Einfluß von Hämodilution mit Plasmaproteinlösung und Hydroxyäthylstärke auf das Plasmafibronectin. Anästh Intensivther Notfallmed 19, 175–178, 1984
Kiesewetter H, Jung F, Blume J, Bulling B, Franke RP: Vergleichende Untersuchung von niedermolekularen Dextran- oder Hydroxyäthylstärkelösungen als Volumenersatzmittel bei Hämodilutionstherapie. Klin Wschr 64, 29–37, 1986
Kiesewetter H, Jung F, Blume J, Gerhards M: Hämodilution bei Patienten mit peripherer arterieller Verschlußkrankheit im Stadium IIb: Prospektiver randomisierter Doppelblind-Vergleich von mittelmolekularer Hydroxyäthylstärke und kleinmolekularer Dextranlösung. Klin Wschr 65, 324–330, 1987

Kiesewetter H, Radtke H, Schneider R, Mussler K, Scheffler A, Schmid-Schönbein H: Das Mini-Erythro-zytenaggregometer: Ein neues Gerät zur schnellen Quantifizierung des Ausmaßes der Ery-throzytenaggregation. Biomed Technik 27, 209–213, 1982

Kiesewetter H, Waldhausen P, Schimetta W, Wilhelm H-J, Koscielny J: Possible side effects of a HES in-fusion and their treatment. In: Koscielny J, Kiesewetter H, Jung F, Haaß A (eds) Hemodilution. New aspects in the management of circulatory blood flow. Improvement of macro- and microcirculation. Springer, Berlin Heidelberg New York, 165–170, 1992

Kline RA, Negendank W, McCoy L, Berguer R: Benefical effects of isovolemic hemodilution using perflurocarbon emulsion in a stroke model. Am J Surg 162, 103–106, 1991

Köhler H, Zschiedrich H, Clasen R, Linfante A, Gamm H: Blutvolumen, kolloidosmotischer Druck und Nierenfunktion von Probanden nach Infusion von mittelmolekularer 10% Hydroxyäthylstärke 200/0,5 und 10% Dextran 40. Anaesthesist 31, 61–67, 1982

Köhler K, Zschiedrich H, Linfante A, Appel F, Pitz H, Clasen R: Die Elimination von Hydroxyäthylstärke 200/0,5, Dextran 40 und Oxypolygelatine. Klin Wschr 60, 293–301, 1982

Koscielny J, Förster H, Kolepke W, Jung F: Vergleich von iso- und hypervolämischer Hämodilution mit HES. In: Koscielny J, Kiesewetter H, Jung F, Haaß A (Hrsg): Hämodilution, neue Aspekte in der Behandlung von Durchblutungsstörungen. Springer, Berlin Heidelberg New Nork, 146–228, 1991

Költringer P, Pfeiffer KP, Lind P, Wakonig P, Langsteger W, Eber O, Reisecker F: Hämodilution mit mittelmolekularer Hydroxyäthylstärke - 6% HÄS 200000/0,60–0,66 - bei Patienten mit peripherer arterieller Verschlußkrankheit. Österreichische Krankenhauspharmazie 3, 7–12, 1989

Krentzlin M, Sens B, Barthels M: Subnormale Ristocetin Cofaktor-Werte (VIIIR:RCF) und Blu-tungsbereitschaft. In: Landbeck G (Hrsg) 16. Hämophilie Symposion, Hamburg. Springer, Berlin Heidelberg New York, 207–209, 1985

Kristensen SD, Milner PC, Martin JF: Bleeding time and platelet volume in acute myocardial infarction. A 2 year follow-up study. Thromb Haemost 59, 353–356, 1988

Kroemer H, Haaß A, Müller K, Jäger H, Wagner EM, Heimburg P, Klotz U: Haemodilution therapy in ischaemic stroke: plasma concentrations and plasma viskosity during long-term infusion of dex-tran 40 or hydroxyethyl starch 200/0,5. Eur J Clin Pharmacol 31, 705–710, 1987

Lackner F, Graninger W, Khosropour R: Senkt Gelatine als Blutersatzmittel selektiv das Plasmafibronectin ? Anaesthesist 34, 470–473, 1985

Landgraf H, Ehrly AM, Saeger-Lorenz K, Vogel C: Untersuchung über den Einfluß einer Infusion von mittelmolekularer Hydroxyäthylstärke (HES-steril 10%) auf die Fließeigenschaften des Blutes gesunder Probanden. Infusionstherapie 4, 200–204, 1981

Lang C: Risiken und Nebenwirkungen der Hämodilutionstherapie. Nervenheilkunde 11, 44–47, 1992

Larrieu MJ, Weiland C: Utilisation de la "cephaline" dans les testes de coagulation. Rev Hemat 12, 199–210, 1957

Lee R, Neya K, Svizzero TA, Vlahakes GJ: Limitations of the efficacy of hemoglobin-based oxygen-carring solutions. J Appl Physiol 79, 236–242, 1995

Lenz G, Hempel V, Junger H, Werle H, Buckenmaier P: Auswirkungen von Hydroxyäthylstärke, Oxy-polygelatine und Humanalbumin auf die Phagozytosefunktion des Retikuloendothelialen Systems (RES) gesunder Probanden. Anaesthesist 35, 423–428, 1986

Leonov Y, Sterz F, Safar P, Johnson DW, Tisherman SA, Oku K: Hypertension with hemodilution prevents multifocal cerebral hypoperfusion after cardiac arrest in dogs. Stroke 23, 45–53, 1992

Levin J, Bessman JD: The inverse relation between platelet volume and platelet number. J Lab Clin Med 101, 295–307, 1983

Lin S-Z, Chiou T-L, Chiang Y-H, Song W-S: Hemodilution accelerates the passage of plasma (not red cells) through cerebral microvessels in rats. Stroke 26, 2166–2171, 1995

Lockwood DNJ, Bullen C, Machin SJ: A severe coagulophathy following volume replacement with hydroxyethylstarch in a jehovahs witness. Anaesthesia 43, 391–393, 1988

London MJ, Ho JS, Triedman JK, Verrier ED, Levine J, Merrick SH, Hanley FL, Browner WS, Mangono DT: A randomized clinical trial of 10% pentastarch (low molecular weight hydroxyethyl starch) versus 5% albumine for plasma volume expansion after cardiac operations. J Thorac Cardiovasc Surg 97, 785–797, 1989

Lukowsky A, Mielke F: Zur Rolle von Fibronectin bei der unspezifischen Abwehr aus immunologischer Sicht. Z Gesamte Inn Med 41, 437–440, 1986

Lundsgaard-Hansen P, Doran JE, Rubli E: Die akutmedizinische Relevanz von Plasma-Fibronectin. Folia Haematol Leipzig 113, 435–445, 1986

Matsui T, Sinyama H, Asano T: Benefical effect of prolonged administration of albumine on ischemic cerebral edema and infarction after occlusion of middle cerebral artery in rats. Neurosurgery 33, 293–300, 1993

Messmer K, Jesch F: Volumenersatz und Hämodilution durch Hydroxyäthylstärke. Infusionstherapie 5, 169–177, 1978

Mishler JM: Pharmakokinetik mittelmolekularer Hydroxyäthylstärke (HÄS 200/0,5). Infusionstherapie 7, 96–102, 1980

Molendijk L, Malburg I, Kopecky P: Dopplersonographische Untersuchungen bei Plazentainsuffizienz als Hinweis auf die Effektivität der Hämodilutionstherapie. Z Geburtshilfe Perinatol 199, 18–22, 1995

Mork T, Hancock REW: Mechanisms of nonopsonic phagocytosis of pseudomonas aeroginosa. Infect Immun 61, 3287–3293, 1993

Mosher DF, Furcht LT: Fibronectin: Review of its structure and possible functions. J Invest Dermatol 77, 175–180, 1981

Olsen TS, Larsen B, Herning M, Skriver EB, Lassen NA: Blood flow and vascular reactivity in collaterally perfused brain tissue. Evidence of an ischemic penumbra in patients with acute stroke. Stroke 14, 332–341, 1983

Olsen TS: Regional cerebral blood flow after occlusion of the middle cerebral artery. Acta Neurol Scand 73, 321–337, 1986

Pearlstein E, Gold LI, Garcia-Pardo A: Fibronectin: a review of its structure and biological activity. Mol Cell Biochem 29, 103–128, 1980

Pelzer H, Schwarz A, Heimburger N: Enzyme immunoassay for determination of human thrombin/antithrombin III complex. Thromb Research, Suppl. VI, 51, 1986

Peter K, Gander HP, Lutz H, Nold W, Strosiek U: Die Beeinflussung der Blutgerinnung durch Hydroxyäthylstärke. Anaesthesist 24, 219–224, 1975

Popov-Cenic S, Müller N, Kladetzky R-G, Hack G, Lang U, Safer A, Rahlfs VW: Durch Prämedikation, Narkose und Operation bedingte Änderungen des Gerinnungs- und Fibrinolysesystems und der Thrombozyten. Einfluß von Dextran und Hydroxyäthylstärke (HÄS) während und nach Operation. Anaesthesist 26, 77–84, 1977

Powell FS, Doran JE: Current status of Fibronectin in transfusion medicine: focus on clinical studies. Vox Sang 60, 193–202, 1991

Rackow EC, Mecher C, Astiz ME, Griffel M, Falk JL, Weil MH: Effects of pentastarch and albumin infusion on cardiorespiratory function and cogulation in patients with severe sepsis and systemic hypoperfusion. Crit Care Med 17, 394–398, 1989

Ramm B, Hofmann G: Biomathematik, Enke, Stuttgart 1987

Ratliff TL, McCarthy R, Telle WB, Brown EJ: Purification of a mycobacterial adhesis to fibronectin. Infect Immun 61, 1889–1894, 1993

Remky A, Wolf S, Hamid M, Bertram B, Schulte K, Arend O, Reim M: Einfluß der Hämodilution auf die retinale Hämodynamik bei Venenastverschlüssen. Ophthalmologe 91, 288–292, 1994

Ringelstein EB, Mauckner A, Schneider R, Sturm W, Doering W, Wolf S, Maurin N, Willmes K, Schlenker M, Brückmann H, Eschenfelder V: Effects of enzymatic blood defibrination in subcortical arteriosclerotic enzephalopathy. J Neurol Neurosurg Psychiat 51, 1051–1057, 1988

Ruggeri ZM, Zimmerman TS: The complex multimeric composition of factor VIII / von Willebrand factor. Blood 57, 1140–1143, 1981

Ruggeri ZM: Pathogenesis and classification of von Willebrand disease. Haemostasis 24, 265–275, 1994

Saba TM, DiLuzio NR: Reticuloendothelial blockade recovery as a function of opsonic activity. Am J Physiol 216, 197–205, 1969

Saba TM, Cho E: Reticuloendothelial systemic response to operative trauma as influenced by cryoprecipitate or cold insoluble globuin therapy. J Reticuloendothel Soc 26, 171–186, 1979

Sanfelippo MJ, Suberviola PD, Geimer NF: Development of a von Willebrand like syndrom after prolonged use of hydroxyethyl starch. Am J Clin Pathol 88, 653–655, 1987

Scheffler P, Jung F, Mrowietz C, Waldhausen P, Leipnitz G, Häuser B: Hämorheologische, mikro- und makrozirkulatorische Effekte einer hypervolämischen Infusion mittelmolekularer Hydroxyäthylstärke (10%, 200000/0,62) bei Gesunden. Infusionstherapie 14, 233–238, 1987

Schildt B, Bouveng R, Sollenberg M: Plasma substitute induced impairment of the reticuloendothelial system function. Acta Chir Scand 141, 7–13, 1975

Schlegelberger B, Plendl H, Grote W: Die Bestimmung von Faktor VIIIR:AG. Vergleich zwischen Enzymimmunoassay und Immunelektrophorese. in: Roka L, Spanuth E (Hrsg) Neue Aspekte in der Gerinnungsdiagnostik. Schattauer, Stuttgart-New York, 121–128, 1984

Shatney CH, Chaudry IH: Hydroxyethylstarch administration does not depress reticuloendothelial function or increase mortality from sepsis. Circ Shock 13, 21–26, 1984

Shoemaker WC, Kram HB: Effects of crystalloids and colloids on hemodynamics, oxygen transport and outcome in high-risk surgical patients. in: Simmons RC, Udekuo AS (eds) Debates in clinical surgery. Yearbook, Chicago 263–316, 1990

Siostrzonek P, Niessner H, Deutsch E, Lechner K, Korninger C, Pabinger I, Heinz R: Vier Fälle mit erworbenem von Willebrand-Syndrom und monoklonaler Gammopathie. Langzeitverlauf sowie diagnostische und therapeutische Problematik. In: Landbeck G (Hrsg) 16. Hämophilie Symposion, Hamburg. Springer, Berlin Heidelberg New York, 248–256, 1985

Schmid-Schönbein H: Physiologie und Pathophysiologie der Mikrozirkulation aus rheologischer Sicht. Internist 23, 359–374, 1982

Sommermeyer K, Cech F, Schmidt M, Weidler B: Klinisch verwendete Hydroxyethylstärke: physikalisch-chemische Charakterisierung. Krankenhauspharmazie 8, 271–278, 1987

Spahn DR: New therapeutic concepts using artifical oxygen carriers. In: Baron JF, Treib J (eds) Volume Replacement. Springer Berlin, Heidelberg, New York, 121–133, 1998

Spence RK: Perfluocarbons in the twenty-first century: Clinical applications as transfusion alternatives. Art Cell Blood Subs and Immob Biotech 23, 367–380, 1995

Staedt U: Hämorheologische, makro- und mikrozirkulatorische Parameter einschließlich ihrer Interaktionen bei Patienten mit akutem Hirninfarkt unter pathophysiologischen und therapeutischen Gesichtspunkten. Habilitationsschrift, Heidelberg, 1994

Strauss RG, Stansfield C, Henriksen RA, Villhauer PJ: Pentastarch may cause fewer effects on coagulation than hetastarch. Transfusion 28, 257–260, 1988

Stump DC, Strauss RG, Henriksen RA, Petersen RE, Saunders R: Effects of hydroxyethyl starch on blood coagulation, particularly factor VIII. Transfusion 25, 349–354, 1985

Symington BE: Hetastarch and bleeding complications. Ann Intern Med 105, 627–628, 1986

Szepfalusi Z, Parth E, Jurecka W, Luger TA, Kraft D: Human monocytes and keratinocytes in culture ingest hydroxyethylstarch. Arch Dermatol Res 285, 144–150, 1993

Thompson CB, Eaton KA, Princiotta SM, Rushin CA, Valeri CR: Size dependent platelet subpopulations: relationship of platelet volume to ultrastructure, enzymatic activity and function. Br J Haematol 50, 509–519, 1982

Thompson WL, Fukushima T, Rutherford RB, Walton RP: Intravasale Persistenz, Gewebsspeicherung und Ausscheidung von Hydroxyäthylstärke (HÄS). Infusionstherapie 6, 151–155, 1979

Threatte GA: Usefulness of the mean platelet volume. Clin Lab Med 13, 937–950, 1993

Treib J, Haaß A, Pindur G, Seyfert UT, Treib W, Grauer MT, Jung F, Wenzel E, Schimrigk K: HES 200/0,5 is not HES 200/0,5. Influence of the C2/C6 hydroxyethylation ratio of hydroxyethyl starch (HES) on hemorheology, coagulation and elimination kinetics. Thromb Haemost 74, 1452–1456, 1995

Treib J, Haaß A, Pindur G, Grauer MT, Wenzel E, Schimrigk K: Abnahme des Thrombozytenvolumens durch mehrtägige Infusion von hochsubstituierter mittelmolekularer Hydroxyäthylstärke (HÄS 200/0,62). Wiener Klinische Wochenschrift 108, 20–23, 1996

Treib J, Haaß A, Pindur G, Treib W, Wenzel E, Schimrigk K: Influence on intravascular molecular weight of hydroxyethyl starch on platelets during a long-term hemodilution. European Journal of Hematology 56, 168–172, 1996

Treib J, Haaß A, Pindur G, Grauer MT, Wenzel E, Schimrigk K: Decrease of fibronectin following repeated infusion of highly substituted hydroxyethyl starch. Infusionstherapie und Transfusionsmedizin 23, 71–75, 1996

Treib J, Haaß A, Pindur G, Grauer MT, Wenzel E, Schimrigk K: All medium starches are not the same: Influence of degree of substitution of hydroxyethyl starch on volumen effect, hemorheologic conditions and coagulation. Transfusion 36, 450–455, 1996

Treib J, Haaß A, Pindur G, Miyachita C, Grauer MT, Jung F, Wenzel E, Schimrigk K: Highly substituted hydroxyethyl starch (HES 200/0.62) leads to a type I von Willebrand syndrome after repeated administration. Haemostasis 26, 210–213, 1996

Treib J, Haaß A, Pindur G: Hetastarch coagulopathy. Journal of Neurosurgery 85, 367–368, 1996

Treib J, Haaß A, Grauer MT, Stoll M, Koch D, Schimrigk K: Comparison of hypervolemic hemodilution concepts in acute stroke. Clinical Hemorheology 16, 367–375, 1996

Treib J, Haaß A, Pindur G, Grauer MT, Seyfert UT, Treib W, Wenzel E, Schimrigk K: Influence of low molecular weight hydroxyethyl starch on hemostasis and hemorheology. Haemostasis 26, 258–265, 1996

Treib J, Haaß A, Pindur G, Treib W, Wenzel E, Schimrigk K: Influence of low and medium molecular weight hydroxyethyl starch on platelets during a long-term hemodilution. Arzneimittelforschung/Drug Research 46, 1064–1066, 1996

Treib J, Haaß A: Hydroxyethyl starch. Journal of Neurosurgery 86, 574–575, 1997

Treib J, Haaß A, Pindur G, Grauer MT, Treib W, Wenzel E, Schimrigk K: Increased hemorrhagic risk after repeated infusion of highly substituted medium molecular weight hydroxyethyl starch (10% HES 200/0.62). Arzneimittelforschung/Drug Research 47, 18–22, 1997

Treib J, Haaß A, Pindur G, Grauer MT, Wenzel E, Schimrigk K: A more differentiated classification of hydroxyethyl starch is nessessary. Intensive Care Medicine 23, 709–710, 1997

Treib J, Haaß A, Pindur G: Coagulation disorders caused by hydroxyethyl starch. Thrombosis and Haemostasis 78, 974–983, 1997

Treib J, Haaß A, Pindur G, Wenzel E, Schimrigk K: Blutungskomplikationen durch Hydroxyethylstärke sind vermeidbar. Deutsches Ärzteblatt 94, 2326–2330, 1997

Treib J, Haaß A, Schimrigk K: European hydroxyethyl starch: a safe and inexpensive alternative to albumine. Anesthesia and Analgesia 85, 709, 1997

Treib J, Haaß A: Rheologische Eigenschaften von Hydroxyethylstärke. Deutsche Medizinische Wochenschrift 122, 1319–1322, 1997

Treib J, Haaß A, Schmid-Schönbein H, Fröhlig G: Bedeutung der Hämodynamik beim akuten Hirninfarkt. Deutsches Ärzteblatt, 96, 553–556, 1999

Treib J, Baron JF, Grauer MT, Strauss RG. An International View of Hydroxyethyl starches. Intensive Care Medicine, 25, 258–268, 1999

Treib J, Haaß A: Prävention des Hirninfarktes. Deutsches Ärzteblatt 1999, in press

Treib W: Beeinflussung von Hämorheologie und Gerinnungssystem durch 10% Hydroxyethylstärke (HES) 200/0,5 und 6% 40/0,50–0,55 im Verlauf einer Langzeithämodilutionsbehandlung. Dissertation, Homburg, 1–187, 1993

Trumble ER, Muizelaar JP, Myseros JS, Choi SC, Warren BB: Coagulopathy with the use of hetastarch in the treatment of vasospasm. J Neurosurg 82, 44–47, 1995

Vinazzer H, Bergmann H: Zur Beeinflussung postoperativer Änderungen der Blutgerinnung durch Hydroxyäthylstärke. Anaesthesist 24, 517–520, 1975

Waxman K, Holness R, Tominaga G, Chela P, Grimes J: Hemodynamic and oxygen transport effects of pentastarch in burn resuscitaion. Ann Surg 209, 341–345, 1989

Witzleb E: Viskosität in Blutgefäßen. in: Schmidt F, Thews G (Hrsg) Physiologie des Menschen. Springer, Berlin Heidelberg New York Tokio 436–437, 1985

Xie DL, Meyers R, Homandberg GA: Release of elastase from monocytes adherent to fibronectin-gelatin surface. Blood 81, 186–192, 1992

Yang KD, Augustine NH, Shaio M-F, Bohnsack JF, Hill HR: Effects of fibronectin on actin organization and respiratory burst activity in neutrophils, monocytes, and macrophages. J Cellular Physiology 158, 347–353, 1994

Yoshida M, Yamashita T, Matsuo J, Kishikawa T: Enzymic degradation of hydroxyethyl starch. Part I. Influence of the distribution of hydroxyethyl groups on the enzymic degradation of hydroxyethyl starch. Stärke 25, 373–376, 1973

Yoshida M, Kishikawa T: A study of hydroxyethyl starch. Part II. Degradation-sites of hydroxyethyl starch by pig pankreas alpha-amylase. Starch/Stärke 36, 167–169, 1984

Yoshida M, Minami Y, Kishikawa T: A study of hydroxyethyl starch. Part III. Comparison of metabolic fates between 2-o-hydroxyethyl starch and 6-o-hydroxyethyl starch in rabbits. Starch/Stärke 36, 209–212, 1984

Zimmerman TS, Ruggeri ZM: Von Willebrand's Disease. Clin Haematol 12, 175–200, 1983

CHAPTER 8

Hydroxyethyl Starch and Reperfusion Injury

R. SCHELL, G. STIER, D. J. COLE

Introduction

"Blood...appears to carry life to every part of the body, for whenever, the whole or a part is deprived of fresh blood it very soon dies" [1]. This statement, made in the early 19th century seems intuitively obvious; and indeed has served as a foundation of clinical management of ischemia – *restore perfusion*. However, in the last decade it has become apparent that re-establishment of blood flow to ischemic tissue not only restores energy supply and removes toxic metabolites but, paradoxically, may worsen the original ischemic injury [2]. Free radical formation, release of inflammatory mediators, and capillary leakiness may result [3–6]. Most of the attempts to restore microvascular function have been directed at the prevention or correction of biochemical aberrations that occur during ischemia or on reperfusion. Clinical examples of potential reperfusion injury are demonstrated in Table 1.

Recently, investigation has focused on the potential of hydroxyethyl starch (HES) as a resuscitative fluid for temporary organ ischemia with reperfusion. Hydroxyethyl starch is available commercially as solutions with a wide range of molecular weights, or experimentally as more narrow molecular weight fractions.

The interendothelial junction forms a primary component of the blood-tissue barrier. This barrier acts to preserve intravascular fluid volume and restrict extravasation of intravascular proteins, polar solutes, and the attendant volume into the interstitial space. However following a period of transient ischemia these interendothelial junctions "open"; thus allowing "third spacing" of intravascular volume and vasogenic edema which often contributes to the ultimate injury [7–10]. Accordingly, fluid resuscitation during periods of increased microvascular permeability represent a conflict between restoration of intravascular volume without unnecessary accumulation of extravascular fluid. This concept is mathematically represented by the Starling equation for microvascular fluid flux:

$$Q_f = L_p A \left[(P_{mv} - P_i) + \sigma(\pi_i - \pi_p) \right]$$

where Q_f=the rate of fluid filtration out of the capillary bed, L_p=the hydraulic con-

Table 1. Clinical examples of reperfusion injury with altered microvascular permeability

Heart	Myocardial ischemia/infarction, transplantation
Kidney	Renal ischemia during aortic crossclamp, transplantation
Skeletal Muscle	Tourniquet use, crush injuries, vascular injuries
Brain	Stroke, cardiac arrest, traumatic injury
Spinal Cord	Thoracic aortic crossclamp, traumatic
Lung	Endotoxemia, adult respiratory distress syndrome, transplantation
GI Tract	Shock, occlusion of mesenteric vessels
Thermal Injury	Burns, hypothermia

ductivity of the microvascular barrier, A=the microvascular surface area, P_{mv}= microvascular hydrostatic pressure, P_i=interstitial hydrostatic pressure, σ=the reflection coefficient for plasma proteins, $π_i$=interstitial colloid osmotic pressure, and $π_p$=plasma colloid osmotic pressure. Thus, strategies to keep fluid in the vascular space would focus on decreasing microvascular hydrostatic pressure, increasing plasma colloid osmotic pressure, and decreasing capillary permeability [11].

An intravenous fluid that expands intravascular volume and also minimizes leakage of fluid into the interstitium would be ideal. We will briefly review the pathophysiology of reperfusion injury and discuss the possible mechanisms and current evidence for a beneficial role for HES in reducing reperfusion injury.

Pathophysiology of Ischemia and Reperfusion

Pathophysiologic metabolic pathways (simplified) involved during ischemia and reperfusion [3] are demonstrated in figure 1. With ischemia, the production of adenosine triphosphate (ATP) is greatly reduced or absent, but the use of ATP continues. ATP is sequentially broken down into adenosine monophosphate, adenosine, inosine, and hypoxanthine. Anaerobic glycolysis, ionic pump failure, and activation of N-methyl-D-Aspartate (NMDA) receptors leads to intracellular acidosis and increased intracellular calcium. The enzyme xanthine dehydrogenase (the predominant form of the enzyme in healthy cells) is altered to function as xanthine oxidase (XO) by a calcium activated intracellular protease.

With reperfusion and reintroduction of oxygen, there are several major mechanisms instrumental in the development of postischemic injury. Oxygen free radicals (superoxide radical, hydrogen peroxide, and hydroxyl radical) are unstable, highly reactive molecules which cause injury to proteins, lipids, and nucleic acids. Although oxygen radicals are normally produced in relatively small amounts under aerobic conditions, they are inactivated by endogenous free radical scavengers (superoxide dismutase, catalase). Radical production can occur by pathways in both parenchyma and vascular endothelium and are produced in excess during reperfusion. Hypoxanthine, which accumulates during ischemia, is metabolized with oxygen by XO into xanthine with oxygen as an electron acceptor producing superoxide radical and hydrogen peroxide. The superoxide anion can reduce ferric ion (Fe^{+3}) regenerating ferrous ion (Fe^{+2}) which can catalyze the formation of hydroxyl radicals. Polyunsaturated fatty acids present in cell membranes are particularly susceptible to reactions with oxygen radicals. The presence of hydroxyl radical, especially in the setting of tissue acidosis, results in lipid peroxidation within the cellular membranes causing loss of membrane structure and function. Lipid peroxidation in the vascular endothelium causes increased microvascular permeability. Enhanced neutrophil adesion to endothelium occurs in postcapillary venules during ischemia with a more pronounced effect during reperfusion. Activated neutrophils adhere to and migrate across the endothelium and release free radicals and destructive proteolytic enzymes (elastase, collagenase) causing local and systemic damage. Cellular phospholipase activity (stimulated by intracellular calcium) is increased which stimulates arachnidonic acid metabolism with concomitant production of oxygen radicals, pros-

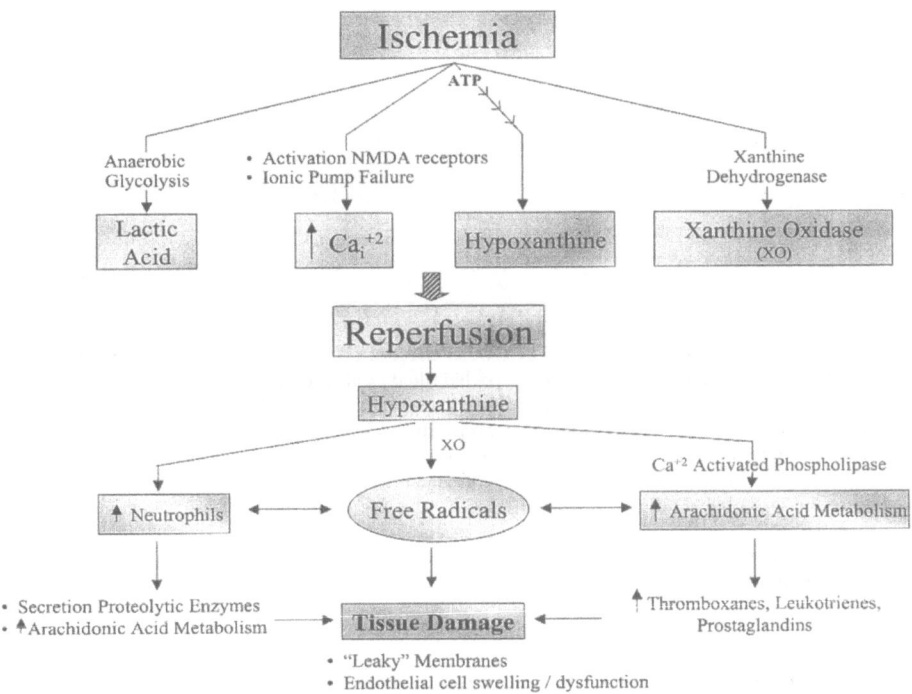

Fig. 1. A simplified flow diagram of several of the major metabolic pathways involved during ischemia and reperfusion. (Ca^{+2}_i = intracellular calcium)

taglandins, thromboxanes, and leukotrienes which may increase microvascular permeability, alter microvascular fluid flow, and recruit additional granulocytes.

Mechanisms by Which HES Might Reduce Reperfusion Injury

Hydroxyethyl starch has been demonstrated to reduce reperfusion injury in many animal models and organ systems [7, 12–19]. Mechanisms proposed to explain HES mediated tissue protection are demonstrated in Figure 1 and include a "capillary sealant" effect that decreases tissue edema, reduced neutrophil adherence to endothelial cells potentially decreasing neutrophil-mediated oxidant injury, a free radical scavenging effect especially when conjugated with deferoxamine, oncotic effects, antiinflammatory properties, and an improvement in blood rheology.

There remains considerable clinical and experimental controversy regarding the efficacy of colloidal solutions in resuscitation and fluid management under various pathophysiologic states, including ischemia with reperfusion. The crystalloid-colloid controversy will not be discussed in this review. The question, however, is HES just another colloidal fluid like albumin or are there unique properties of HES that would

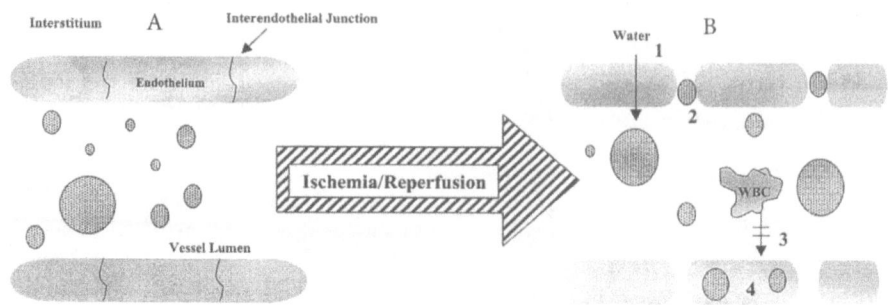

Fig. 2A,B. Proposed mechanisms for a beneficial effect of HES on cellular injury following a period of tissue ischemia and reperfusion. The speckled filled circles represent different sizes of HES molecules. **A.** Represents the normal state with relatively tight interendothelial junctions. **B.** Represents the proposed state after ischemia and during reperfusion. #1 indicates a favorable oncotic effect of intravascular HES which acts to attract water from the extravascular space into the vessel lumen. #2 represents HES acting as a physical sealant at separated interendothelial junctions. #3 conveys a reduced neutrophil-endothelial cell interaction with an effective decreased oxidant injury. #4 indicates a physical sealant effect of HES at the microvascular matrix barrier. Other possible mechanisms not demonstrated include a rheological effect, and an effect at the endothelial glycocalyx to decrease resistance to blood flow.

support their use not only for maintenance of intravascular volume but also for a therapeutic "drug" effect in the scenario of ischemia with reperfusion?

Reduction in Microvascular "Leakiness"

One of the pathologic results of ischemia with reperfusion is microvasculature "leakiness". The process of vasculature leak is primarily the result of endothelial cell contraction and consequent separation of intercellular endothelial cell junctions occuring predominantly in the postcapillary (pericytic) venules, although separation of interendothelial clefts is not a necessary element for increases in microvascular permeability [20–25]. Interstitial or "third space" accumulation of fluid may impair the diffusion of oxygen and energy substrates to the cells and the removal of carbon dioxide and organic acids (lactate). Tissue pressure may be increased resulting in venous congestion. An ideal fluid resuscitation regimen would be expected to limit edema formation at the site of injury by minimizing the impact of a rapid increase in capillary permeability. This resuscitative fluid would remain within the vascular compartment restoring and maintaining normal hemodynamic parameters, restore the selective microvascular permeability characteristics at the site of injury, and would accomplish these effects with minimal side effects or untoward reactions.

Many disadvantages of HES are associated with the heterogeneity of the size of the macromolecules making up the solution. The HES solution may have molecules within a size range of 5,000- >1,000,000 daltons, depending on the preparation [26, 27]. Comparatively, the natural hematogenous colloid, albumin, is homogeneous with a molecular weight (MW) of 69,000 daltons. Each fraction of HES has its own pharmacodynamic profile [27]. The extremely high molecular weight HES species have an increased tendency to stay intravascular rather than leak into the interstitium, create favorable oncotic gradients (interstitium to vasculature), and have a longer half life. Improved retention of colloid in the vascular compartment would reduce the transvascular fluid flux and subsequent accumulation of fluid in the interstitial compartment (edema) and result in a more rapid intravascular volume resuscitation possibly limiting reperfusion injury. The low molecular weight starch molecules do not create effective oncotic gradients and may have an easier time passing through areas of the microvasculature that have become leaky. Transvascular passage of macromolecules during reperfusion may occur through separated endothelial junctions, by increased transcytosis (e.g. vesicular transport, transendothelial channels), as the result of endothelial destruction, or by other mechanism(s).

HES as a Physical Sealant at Separated Interendothelial Junctions

Zikria and others have suggested that "appropriately sized" fractions of HES may actually act as physical plugs at "holes" or separated interendothelial junctions in the microvasculature thereby reducing interstitial edema formation [7, 14, 28, 29]. This has led to laboratory investigations of various MW fractions of HES in an attempt to determine the most beneficial MW size range of HES macromolecules which act to "plug" a leaky microvascular barrier. Most clinical and experimental efforts that address this issue are based on the hypothesis that if one were able to reduce microvascular permeability, reduce the total amount of resuscitation fluid given while simultaneously restoring systemic hemodynamic parameters, then acccumulation of edema fluid would be decreased.

HES as a Physical Sealant of the Microvascular Matrix Barrier

Increased microvascular permeability with extravasation of macromolecules following ischemia with reperfusion may occur without actual separation of the interendothelial junctions [13, 25, 30, 31]. One postulate [17] is that extravasation may result from disorganization in the fiber matrix of the postcapillary venules without separation of endothelial junctions but with reduced function of this microvascular barrier. The HES macromolecules, because of their high molecular weight and large hydrodynamic radius, cross the the fiber matrix at a slower rate, and serve to seal the interstices and restore the macromolecular exchange rate closer to baseline. In this hypothesis, HES would act in a physiochemical way to attenuate microvascular transport dysfunction.

HES and Altered Vesicular Transport

Transcellular vesicular transport of macromolecules may occur via pinocytotic vesicles and transendothelial channels [32]. Although it has been postulated that HES might reduce trancytosis [13], the interaction between HES and transcellular vesicular transport has not been defined.

Reduction in Oxidant Mediated Injury

Oxygen free radical formation with cell damage resulting from lipid peroxidation of cell membranes is an important mechanism of ischemia-reperfusion injury. Neutrophil-endothelial cell interactions are a prerequisite for the microvascular injury induced by ischemia-reperfusion [33]. Activated neutrophils adhere to and migrate across the endothelium and cause local destruction by releasing free radicals and proteolytic enzymes. HES has been shown to scavenge hydroxyl radical in vitro, reduce neutrophil binding to stimulated endothelial cells, and reduce the amount of the oxidant generating enzyme xanthine oxidase [12, 17, 18 34].

Rheologic/Vascular Resistance Changes

Acellular fluids such as HES have a viscosity less than whole blood; thus, facilitating blood flow via improved rheology [35, 36]. Hemodilution is postulated to favorably affect ischemia by augmenting blood flow via three mechanisms [37, 38]. The first mechanism is by decreasing viscosity, of which hematocrit is the major determinant; while the second is a direct myogenic vasodilatory response to a reduction in oxygen content. The third mechanism is postulated to occur by an action of the hemodiluent to remove plasma proteins which are adsorbed at the endothelial glycocalyx. The adsorbed proteins result in a thickened glycocalyx and act to impede flow at the luminal surface.

Current Evidence Regarding HES and Reperfusion Injury

Central Nervous System

Hydroxyethyl starch has been investigated in the setting of focal [13] and global cerebral ischemia [39], spinal cord ischemia [7], and blood-brain [40] and blood-retinal barrier [41, 42] disruption. During cerebral reperfusion there is a transient but profound increase in blood-brain barrier (BBB) permeability that can effect an extensive worsening of brain edema [9]. Schell et al. [13] in a rat model of temporary middle cerebral artery occlusion compared the effects of hemodilution to a hematocrit of 30% with pentastarch versus albumin. Although albumin and pentastarch have a similar osmotic and oncotic pressure, pentastarch reduced BBB permeability, brain edema, and brain injury. Even though a mechanical "plugging" of pentastarch at the interendothelial tight junction could not be demonstrated, the presence of multiple pinocytotic vesicles and transendothelial channels in the electron micrographs suggested a functional effect of pentastarch on BBB permeability. It was postulated that pentastarch reduced vasogenic edema by reducing transcytosis of serum proteins.

In a model using hyperosmolar mannitol to disrupt the BBB in rats, Chi et al. [40] compared hemodilution with lactated Ringer's solution, hetastarch, or a fraction of HES macromolecules (HES-Pz, MW≈100,000–1,000,000 daltons) and demonstrated that HES-Pz was effective in preventing BBB disruption. In a rabbit model of transient spinal cord ischemia, HES-Pz reduced microvascular permeability, neuronal membrane injury, and the incidence of paraplegia as compared to normal saline and HES [7]. The iron chelator deferoxamine (DFO) has been conjugated to HES and evaluated in a cat ischemia-reperfusion model of retinal ischemia [41]. Iron is important in initiating and catalyzing free radical reactions causing oxygen dependent tissue injury. The DFO-HES conjugate lacks vascular permeability and is limited to the vasculature. Gehlbach et al. [41] demonstrated a protective effect of the HES-DFO conjugate on the blood-retinal barrier.

Conversely, Goulin et al. [39] in a rabbit model of global cerebral ischemia with reperfusion utilized normal saline, pentastarch, or hypertonic saline to hemodilute the animals to a hematocrit of 20%. No decrease in brain water content was associated with the administration of pentastarch and the efficacy of HES in reducing brain edema was questioned in an accompanying editorial [11]. Finally, a clinical trial of pentastarch in acute stroke was terminated because of excess mortality in the treatment group (nine pentastarch vs three control) although methodological/randomization concerns (nearly twice as many patients with severe strokes were randomized to the pentastarch group) were raised [43]. However, there was a beneficial effect of pentastarch in a subgroup of patients that received early hemodilution therapy, and in whom pentastarch resulted in an increase in cardiac output. A more recent clinical trial, the Multicenter Austrian Hemodilution Stroke Trial [44] compared 10% HES against pure rehydration with Ringer's lactate in a study of mild hypervolemic hemodilution (HHD) in stroke. Although fewer patients died in the HHD and slightly more HHD patients had improved function at 3 months, the differences were not statistically significant. The trial was terminated because at least 600 patients per group would have been required for significant results.

A solution of HES contains large, ethylated starch or glucose polymers that are metabolized by serum amylases to produce smaller molecules of starch polymers and free glucose [45]. Of concern is the theoretical potential for HES to induce or potentiate hyperglycemia which may worsen neurologic outcome after cerebral ischemia with reperfusion although limited data has not confirmed this possibility [46]. In addition, in laboratory investigations outside of the CNS, the specific molecular weight range of the HES molecule appears to be critical in determining efficacy. The low MW fractions of HES may pass through the microvasculature possibly worsening interstitial edema and the very large MW fractions may not be effective. Clearly, the use of HES in CNS ischemia with reperfusion merits further laboratory and clinical study.

HES and Microvascular Permeability/Reperfusion Injury Outside the CNS

Fractions of HES macromolecules have been shown to be beneficial in the treatment of ischemia-reperfusion outside of the CNS. Although the mechanism is incompletely understood, the hypothesis that appropriately sized biodegradable HES macromolecules might act as biomolecular plugs, and seal or restore microvascular integrity at capillary-endothelial junctions has considerable support from laboratory investigations in various tissues.

Myocardium

In a canine myocardial ischemia model with reperfusion, Ringer's lactate solution, serum albumin, and HES-Pz (70% of macromolecules between 100,000-1 million daltons) were compared [14]. HES-Pz significantly reduced myocardial water content and infarct size. In a similar model [16]. Oz et al. demonstrated that HES-Pz reduced reperfusion injury. HES-Pz alone and with superoxide dismutase (a free radical scavenger) significantly reduced reperfusion injury although addition of superoxide dismutase to HES-Pz did not have an additive effect. Clinical studies to support or refute a role for HES in myocardial ischemia-reperfusion are lacking.

Skeletal Muscle

Reperfusion of skeletal muscle may result in increased microvascular permeability, edema formation, increased tissue hydrostatic pressure with compression ischemia (compartment syndrome), and muscle necrosis [47]. In a rat limb ischemia-reperfusion model utilizing 2-hours of tourniquet ischemia and reperfusion Zikria et al. [29] evaluated lactated Ringer's solution, serum albumin 5%, or varying MW fractions of HES, glycogen and dextran. After 24 hours of reperfusion, the water content and potassium differences between the ischemic and control gastrocnemius muscles were compared. Rats given a 100,000-300,000 dalton fraction of HES had sgnificantly decreased water content than those receiving lactated Ringer's, smaller MW fractions of HES (<100,000 daltons), <300,000 dalton MW glycogen, or dextran 150,000 dalton MW. The molecular weight fractions 100,000-300,000 daltons and 300,000-1,000,000 daltons, appeared to be the most effective in preventing ischemic muscle edema and necrosis.

Pentafraction 5% (PF), a solution of HES macromolecules with molecular weights of ≈100,000-1,000,000 daltons, was investigated in a rabbit hind limb model of skeletal muscle ischemia [48]. Pentafraction or normal saline was administered during reperfusion. Anterior compartment pressure, quantitative oxidative metabolism, and muscle wet-to-dry weight ratios were assessed. Anterior compartment pressure in the normal saline group increased significantly during reperfusion, whereas it remained essentially unchanged in the PF group. After 2 hours of reperfusion, measures of active oxidative metabolism were significantly better in the PF group suggesting better muscle salvage. However, there was no between groups difference in muscle water content. The authors concluded that PF may "plug" interendothelial clefts at the capillary level but did not have an explanation for the non-supportive dry-to-wet muscle weight ratios.

It is thought that neutrophils may have a role in oxidative injury and no-reflow phenomenon [49, 50]. Oz et al. [17] studied not only the effect of HES macromolecules (HES-Pz fraction) on microvascular permeability in postischemic striated muscle but also attempted to describe the effect of HES-Pz on binding interactions between injured/stimulated endothelial cells and neutrophils. Rat cremasteric muscle was made ischemic for 4-hours and 2-hours of reperfusion allowed. Just prior to re-establishing blood flow, either saline or a 6% solution of HES-Pz was administered in a volume equal to 10% of the animal's blood volume. They demonstrated a beneficial effect of HES-Pz on microvascular transport of macromolecules. Even more interesting, they demonstrated that thrombin stimulated human umbilical vein endothelial cells bound fewer neutrophils when treated with 6% HES-Pz than with saline control. This reduced neutrophil binding to stimulated endothelial cells provides support for another mechanism for HES-Pz influencing reperfusion injury – reduced neutrophil binding to the endothelial surface. The role of leukocytes as injurious in reperfusion injury in skeletal muscle was further elucidated recently in a canine gracilis muscle model [51]. Following 5 hours of ischemia, the treatment muscle was initially reperfused for 40 minutes with blood depleted of leukocytes and several complement factors (resuspended in 5% HES), then 2 days of normal perfusion. They demonstrated reduced muscle necrosis and an improvement in early blood flow. However, the observed decrease in muscle necrosis was not associated with a decrease in edema formation.

Lung

Lung injury may occur after hepatoenteric ischemia (e.g., aortic crossclamping) with reperfusion. An important mechanism is the release of the oxidant-generating enzyme xanthine oxidase (XO) with resultant remote pulmonary injury [52]. Following 40 minutes of aortic occlusion with 3-hours of reperfusion in rabbits using either lactated Ringer's solution or HES (6% pentastarch containing balanced electrolytes), Axon et al [12] demonstrated significantly decreased remote pulmonary injury with the HES solution and decreased release of XO. They previously had demonstrated that HES had a better effect on remote lung injury than 5% albumin or lactated Ringer's. However, both colloidal solutions, and not just the HES reduced gastric injury and XO release after hepatoenteric ischemia-reperfusion [34].

Oxygen-derived free radicals have been implicated in the pathogenesis of lung injury after cardiopulmonary bypass (CPB). In sheep, Stamler et al [53] examined the effects of priming the CPB pump with a pentastarch solution (PS), PS conjugated to the iron chelator deferoxamine (DFO), or lactated Ringer's solution on lung injury. The oncotic agent PS ameliorated the lung derangements seen after CPB as compared with lactated Ringer's solution. The PS-DFO conjugate however did not provide any additional benefit.

Sepsis is associated with increased capillary permeability in the systemic vasculature including the lungs [54,55]. Solutions of HES appear to be well retained in the circulation during sepsis, may ameliorate the progression of microvascular and parenchymal injury, and may be advantageous when infused chronically to maintain intravascular volume [56–58].

Special Clinical Scenarios and Other Organ Systems

HES has been investigated in resuscitation of hemorrhagic shock [59,60], thermal injury with beneficial [61] or little [62] effect on microcirculatory permeability, intestinal ischemic shock [63], isolated jejunal loop studies [28], and as one component of solutions for simple cold storage or machine perfusion for organ preservation and protection against reperfusion injury prior to kidney, pancreas, heart, lung and liver transplantation [64–68].

HES-Deferoxamine Conjugates

Recently, much emphasis has been placed on the role of iron as a catalyst in the formation of the hydroxyl radical– implicated as a mediator in reperfusion injury. Deferoxamine (DFO), a specific iron chelator, has been shown to inhibit the formation of hydroxyl radicals by removing iron from the oxidation-reduction cyle. Covalently linking DFO to biocompatible high molecular-weight polymers such as HES has decreased the toxicity, increased the half-life, yet maintained the iron chelating properties of the free drug [69]. This complex has been investigated, with favorable results, in models of early sepsis, [70] retinal injury [41,42], myocardial ischemia-reperfusion [71–73], kidney hypoxia/reoxygenation [74], smoke inhalation injury [75], lung injury after CPB [53], hemorrhagic shock [76], hepatic reperfusion [77], and brain ischemia-reperfusion [78].

HES and Small Volume Resuscitation

Limited data on small volume resuscitation with hypertonic solutions (hypertonic saline/hydroxyethyl starch combination) has generated positive results [79,80]. Hypertonic saline combined with HES has theoretical advantages for fluid resuscitation in models of ischemia-reperfusion including rapidity of intravascular volume expansion, less volume of fluid administration required with potentially less intracellular and intercellular edema, maintenance of oncotic pressure, and the previously reviewed beneficial effects of HES.

Summary

The intravenous administration of HES in most published models of ischemia-reperfusion and in various organ systems results in a beneficial effect. The mechanism of this beneficial effect is incompletely understood but may be secondary to a reduction in microvascular "leakiness", reduction in oxidant injury, or by a mechanism(s) yet to be elucidated. Whether the results of these laboratory studies can be extrapolated to clinical scenarios of ischemia-reperfusion has not been validated. If the biophysical model for reducing capillary leakiness is correct, determination of the optimal shape and size of a biodegradable macromolecule appropriate for sealing "leaky" endothelium in a variety of tissues under different pathophysiolgic conditions (e.g. shock, organ transplantation, myocardial ischemia, adult respiratory distress syndrome) should be possible. However, until *clinical* studies unequivocally demonstrate a beneficial effect for HES in reducing ischemia-reperfusion injury, it will likely continue to be thought of by most clinicians as just another colloidal fluid to effectively replace intravascular volume.

References

1. Hunter J. Lectures on the principles of surgery. In: Palmer JF, ed. The Works of John Hunter. Vol. 1. London: Longman, 1835:231
2. Parks DA, Granger DN. Contributions of ischemia and reperfusion to mucosal lesion formation. Am J Physiol 1986;250:G749–53
3. Grace PA. Ischaemia-reperfusion injury. Br J Surg 1994;81:637–47
4. Traystman RJ, Kirsch JR, Koehler RC. Oxygen radical mechanisms of brain injury following ischemia and reperfusion. J Appl Physiol 1991;71(4):1185–95
5. Hallenbeck JM, Dutka AJ. Background review and current concepts of reperfusion injury. Arch Neurol 1990;47:1245–54
6. Rubin BB, Romaschin A, Walker PM, et al. Mechanisms of postischemic injury in skeletal muscle: intervention strategies. J Appl Physiol 1996;80(2):369–87
7. Wisselink W, Patetsios P, Panetta TF, Ramirez JA, Rodino W, Kirwin JD, Zikria BA. Medium molecular weight pentastarch reduces reperfusion injury by decreasing capillary leak in an animal model of spinal cord ischemia. J Vasc Surg 1998;27:109–116
8. Cotrina ML, Kang J, Lin JH-C, Bueno E, Hansen TW, He L, Liu Y, Nedergaard M. Astrocytic gap junction remain open during ischemic conditions. J Neurosci 1998;18:2520–2537
9. Cole DJ, Matsumura JS, Drummond JC, Schultz RL, Wong MH. Time and pressure dependent changes in blood-brain barrier permeability after temporary middle cerebral artery occlusion in rats. Acta Neuropathol 82:266–273, 1991
10. Patel PM, Drummond JC, Cole DJ. Induced hypertension during restoration of flow after temporary middle cerebral artery occlusion in the rat: effect on neuronal injury and edema. Surg Neurol 36:195–201, 1991
11. Prough DS, Kramer G. Medium starch please. Anesth Analg 1994;79:1034–1035
12. Axon RN, Baird MS, Lang JD, et al. PentaLyte decreases lung injury after aortic occlusion-reperfusion. Am J Respir Crit Care Med 1998;157:1982–1990
13. Schell RM, Cole DJ, Schultz RL, et al. Temporary Cerebral Ischemia: Effects of Pentastarch or albumin on reperfusion injury. Anesthesiology 1992;77:86–92
14. Zikria BA, Subbarao C, Oz MC, et al. Hydroxyethyl starch macromolecules reduce myocardial reperfusion injury. Arch Surg 1990;125:930–934
15. Webb, AR, Tighe D, Moss RF, et al. Advantages of a narrow-range, medium molecular weight hydroxyethyl starch for volume maintenance in a porcine model of fecal peritonitis. Crit Care Med 1991;19:409–416
16. Oz MC, Zikria BA, McLeod PF, et al. Hydroxyethyl starch macromolecules and superoxide dismutase effects on myocardial reperfusion injury. Am J Surg 1991;162:59–62
17. Oz MC, FitzPatrick MF, Zikria BA, et al. Attenuation of microvascular permeability dysfunction in post-ischemic striated muscle by hydroxyethyl starch. Microvasc Res 1995;50:71–79
18. Pieper GM, Gross GJ, Kalyanaraman B. An ESR study of the nitroxide radical of pentastarch-conjugated deferoxamine. Free Radic Biol Med 1990;9:211–218
19. Mousa SA, Smith RD. Efficacy and safety of deferoxamine conjugated to hydroxyethyl starch. J Cardiovasc Pharm 1992;19:425–429
20. Joris I, Majno G, Ryan GB. Endothelial contraction in vivo: A study of the rat mesentery. Virchos Arch 1972;12:73

21. Horan KL, Adamski SW, Workensh A, et al. Evidence that prolonged histamine suffusions produce transient increases in vascular permeability subsequent to the formation of venular macromolecular leakage sites. Proof of the Majno-Palade hypothesis. Am J Pathol 1986;123:570
22. Joris I, Majno G, Corey EJ, et al. The mechanism of vascular leakage induced by leukotriene E4: endothelial contraction. Am J Pathol 1987;126:19
23. Grega GJ. Role of the endothelial cell in the regulation of microvascular permeability to molecules. Introductory remarks. Fed Proc 1986;45:75
24. Strock PE, Majno GM. Vascular responses to experimental tourniquet ischemia. Surg Gynecol Obstet 1969;129:309
25. Clough G, Michel CC, Phillips ME. Inflammatory changes in permeability and ultrastructure of single vessels in the frog mesenteric circulation. J Phyiol (London) 1988;395:99–114
26. Quon CY. Clinical pharmacokinetics and pharmacodynamics of colloidal plasma volume expanders. J Cardiothorac Anesth 1988;2(Suppl)1:13–23
27. Klotz U, Kroemer H. Clinical pharmacokinetic considerations in the use of plasma expanders. Clin Pharmacokinet 1987;12:123–135
28. Zikria BA, King TC, Stanford J, Freeman HP. A biophysical approach to capillary permeability. Surgery 1989;105:625–31
29. Zikria BA, Subbarao C, Oz MC, et al. Macromolecules reduce abnormal microvascular permeability in rat limb ischemia-reperfusion injury. Crit Care Med 1989;17:1306–1309
30. Suval WD, Duran WN, Boric MP, et al. Assessment of ischemia-reperfusion injury in skeletal muscle by macromolecular clearance. J Surg Res 1987;42:550–59
31. Suval WD, Duran WN, Boric MP, et al. Microvascular transport and endothelial cell alterations preceding skeletal muscle damage in ischmia and reperfusion injury. Am J Surg 1987;154:211–18
32. Watanabe K. Vascular permeability to macromolecules change qualitative inflammation. Jpn J Pharmacol 1985;39:398
33. Welbourn CRB, Goldman G, Paterson IS, et al. Pathophysiology of ischaemia-reperfusion injury: central role of the neutrophil. Br J Surg 1991;78:651–655
34. Nielsen VG, Tan S, Brix AE, et al. Hextend (hetastarch solution) decreases multiple organ injury and xanthine oxidase release after hepatoenteric ischemia-reperfusion in rabbits. Crit Care Med 1997; 25:(9):1565–74
35. Benis AM, Usami S, Chien S. Effect of hematocrit and inertial losses on pressure-flow relations in the isolated hindpaw of the dog. Circ Res 1970;27:1047–1068
36. Cole DJ, Drummond JC, Patel PM, Marcantonio S. Effects of viscosity and oxygen content of cerebral blood flow in ischemic and normal rat brain. J Neurol Sci 1994;124:15–20
37. Harrison MJG. Influence of haematocrit in the cerebral circulation. Cerebrovas Brain Metab Rev 1989;1:55–67
38. Pries AR, Secomb TW, Sperandio M, Gaehtgens P. Blood flow during hemodilution: effect of plasma composition. Cardiovasc Res 1998;37:225–235
39. Goulin GD, Duthie SE, Zornow MH, et al. Global cerebral ischemia: Effects of pentastarch after reperfusion. Anesth Analg 1994;79:1036–42
40. Chi OZ, Lu X, Wei HM. Hydroxyethyl starch solution attenuates blood-brain barrier disruption caused by intracarotid injection of hyperosmolar mannitol in rats. Anesth Analg 1996;83:336–41
41. Gehlbach P, Purple RL. Enhancement of retinal recovery by conjugated deferoxamine after ischemia-reperfusion. Invest Ophthalmol Vis Sci 1994;35:669–676
42. McGorray J, McGorray S, Qi X, Fitzsimmons J, et al. Conjugated deferoxamine reduces blood-brain barrier disruption in experimental optic neuritis. Ophthalmic Res 1994;26(5):310–23
43. The Hemodilution in Stroke Study Group. Hypervolemic hemodilution treatment of acute stroke. Results of a randomized multicenter trial using pentastarch. Stroke 1989;20:317–323
44. Aichner FT, Fazekas F, Brainin M, et al. Hypervolemic hemodilution in ischemic stroke. The multicenter Austrian hemodilution stroke trial (MAHST). Stroke 1998;29:743–749
45. Hulse JD, Yacobi A. Hetastarch: An overview of the colloid and its metabolism. Drug Intell Clin Pharm 1983;17:334–341
46. Hofer RE, Lanier WL. Effect of hydroxyethylstarch solutions on blood glucose concentrations in diabetic and nondiabetic rats. Crit Care Med 1992;20:211–215
47. Rubin BB, Romaschin A, Walker PM. Mechanisms of postischemic injury in skeletal muscle: intervention strategies. J Appl Physiol 1996;80(2):369–387

48. Hakaim AG, Corsetti R, Cho SI. The pentafraction of hydroxyethyl starch inhibits ischemia-induced compartment syndrome. J Trauma 1994;37(1):18–21
49. Jerome SN, Smith CW, Korthuis RJ. CD 18-dependent adherence reactions play an important role in the development of the no-reflow phenomenon. Am J Physiol 1993;264(33):H479–H483
50. Granger D. Role of xanthine oxidase and granulocytes in ischemia-reperfusion injury. Am J Physiol 1988;255:H1269–H1275
51. Rubin B, Tittley J, Chang G, et al. A clinically applicable method for long-term salvage of postischemic skeletal muscle. J Vasc Surg 1991;13:58–68
52. Terada LS, Dormish JJ, Shanley PF, et al. Circulating xanthine oxidase mediates lung neutrophil sequestration after intestinal ischemia-reperfusion. Am J Physiol 1992;263:L394–L401
53. Stamler A, Wang SY, Aguirre DE, et al. Effects of pentastarch-deferoxamine conjugate on lung injury after cardiopulmonary bypass. Circulation 1996;94(9Suppl):II358–63
54. Judges D, Sharkey P, Ceung A, et al. Pulmonary microvascular fluid flux in a large animal model of sepsis: evidence for increased pulmonary endothelial permeability accompanying surgically induced peritonitis in sheep. Surgery 1986;99:222–234
55. Sibbald WJ, Driedger A, Wells GA, et al. The short term effects of increasing plasma colloid osmotic pressure in patients with noncardiac pulmonary edema. Surgery 1983;93:620–633
56. Morisaki H, Bloos F, Keys J, et al. Compared with crystalloid, colloid therapy slow progression of extrapulmonary tissue injury in septic sheep. J Appl Physiol 1994;77(3):1507–1518
57. Webb AR, Tighe D, Moss RF, et al. Advantages of a narrow-range, medium molecular weight hydroxyethyl starch for volume maintenance in a porcine model of fecal peritonitis. Crit Care Med 1991;19:409–416
58. Traber LD, Brazeal BA, Schmitz M, et al. Pentafraction reduces the lung lymph response after endotoxin administration in the ovine model. Circ Shock 1992;36:93–103
59. Nagy KK, Davis J, Duda J, et al. A comparison of pentastarch and lactated Ringer's solution in the resuscitation of patients with hemorrhagic shock. Circ Shock 1993;40:289–294
60. Whitley JM, Prough DS, Brockschmidt JK, et al. Cerebral hemodynamic effects of fluid resuscitation in the presence of an experimental intracranial mass. Surgery 1991;110:514–22
61. Brazeal BA, Honeycutt D, Traber LD, et al. Pentafraction for superior resuscitation of the ovine thermal burn. Crit Care Med 1995;23:332–339
62. Ferrara JJ, Dyess DL, Collins JN, et al. Effects of pentafraction administration on microvascular permeability alterations induced by graded thermal injury. Surgery 1994;115:182–9
63. Wilma CD, Davidson JA, Armstrong JM, et al. Pentafraction-DuPont versus albumin for resuscitation of a lethal intestinal ischemic shock in rats. Circ Shock 1991;33:216–221
64. Neveux N, De Bandt JP, Charrueau C, et al. Deletion of hydroxyethylstarch from University of Wisconsin solution induces cell shrinkage and proteolysis during and after cold storage of rat liver. Hepatology 1997;25(3):678–682
65. Love RB, Conhaim RL, Harms BA. Effects of University of Wisconsin and Euro-Collins solutions on interstitial pulmonary edema in isolated rat lungs. Transplantation 1996;61:1014–1018
66. Arita S, Asano T, Suzuki S, et al. The efficacy of CMH (Collins modified with HES) solution in canine pancreatic graft preservation. Transplantation Proc 1995;27(6):3035–3036
67. Southard JH, van Gulik TM, Ametani MS, et al. Important components of the UW solution. Transplantation 1990; 49(2):251–257
68. Ko W, Zelano JA, Lazenby WD, et al. Compositional analysis of a modified University of Wisconsin solution for extended myocardial preservation. Circulation 1992;86[suppl II]:I-326–I-332
69. Hallaway PE, Eaton JW, Panter SS, et al. Modulation of deferoxamine toxicity and clearance by covalent attachment to biocompatible polymers. Proc Natl Acad Sci USA 1989;86:10108–12
70. Moch D, Schroppel B, Schoenberg MH, et al. Protective effects of hydroxyethyl starch-deferoxamine in early sepsis. Shock 1995;4(6)425–32
71. Maruyama M, Pieper GM, Kalyanaraman B, et al. Effects of hydroxyethyl starch conjugated deferoxamine on myocardial functional recovery following coronary occlusion and reperfusion in dogs. J Cardiovasc Pharm 1991;17:166–175
72. Mousa SA, Ritger RS, Smith RD. Efficacy and safety of deferoxamine conjugated to hydroxyethyl starch. J Cardiovasc Pharm 1992;19:425–429

73. Lesnefsky EJ, Hedlund BE, Hallaway PE, et al. High-dose iron-chelator therapy during reperfusion with deferoxamine–hydroxyethyl starch conjugate fails to reduce canine infarct size. J Cardiovasc Pharm 1990;16:523–528
74. Paller MS, Hedlund BE. Extracellular iron chelators protect kidney cells from hypoxia/reoxygenation. Free Radic Biol Med 1994;17(6):597–603
75. Demling R, LaLonde C, Ikegami K. Fluid resuscitation with deferoxamine hetastarch complex attenuates the lung and systemic response to smoke inhalation. Surgery 1996;19(3):340–8
76. Jacobs DM, Julsrud JM, Bubrick MP. Iron chelation with a deferoxamine conjugate in hemorrhagic shock. J Surg Res 1991;51(6):484–90
77. Colet JM, Cetiner E, Hedlund BE, et al. Assessment of microvascular integrity in the isolated perfused rat liver by contrast-enhanced MRI. Attenuation of reperfusion injury by conjugated deferoxamine. Magn Reson Med 1996;36(5):753–7
78. Rosenthal RE, Chanderbhan R, Marshall G, et al. Prevention of post-ischemic brain lipid conjugated diene production and neurological injury by hydroxyethyl starch-conjugated deferoxamine. Free Radic Biol Med 1992;12(1):29–33
79. Fischer M, Hossmann KA. Volume expansion during cardiopulmonary resuscitation reduces cerebral no-reflow. Resuscitation 1996;32(3):227–40
80. Vollmar B, Lang G, Menger MD, Messmer K. Hypertonic hydroxyethyl starch restores hepatic microvascular perfusion in hemorrhagic shock. Am J Physiol 1994;266:H1927–34

Subject Index